CW01213225

Meditation Yoga

By the Same Author:
**Practical Yoga: A Pictorial Approach
Healing Yourself Through Okidō Yoga**

Meditation Yoga
The Meiso Yoga of Okidō

by Masahiro Oki

JAPAN PUBLICATIONS, INC.

© 1978 by Masahiro Oki
Translated and Edited by David N. Bradshaw

Published by
JAPAN PUBLICATIONS, INC., Tokyo, Japan

Distributed by
JAPAN PUBLICATIONS TRADING COMPANY
200 Clearbrook Road, Elmsford, N.Y. 10053, U.S.A.
1174 Howard Street, San Francisco, Calif. 94103, U.S.A.
P.O.Box 5030 Tokyo International, Tokyo 101-31, Japan

First Edition: April 1978
ISBN 0-87040-435-9
LCCC No. 77-93244

Printed in Japan by Kyodo Printing Co., Ltd.

Editor's Note

Even today, the Oriental mind tends to think holistically. This is the key to understanding *Meditation Yoga*. In the past, the Hua Yen sect of Buddhism in China developed this trait to the utmost as what is now known as the philosophy of totality. According to this way of thought, everything is interconnected by invisible lines of power and relationship. Nothing can be self-existent or separate. Yet, although man is seen as an integral part of the universe, he should not think as a part, but from the point of view of the whole. Only in this way will true personality emerge, for to be fully ourselves, we must think only of others.

This philosophy has very ancient beginnings and has much in common with the ideas of *Samkhya Yoga*. The aim of the Yogic ascesis is nothing less than to homologize man with the Cosmos. The philosophy of totality was transmitted to Japan as early as the Heian Period (794–1185), for Hua Yen was one of six Buddhist philosophical schools established in the capital, Kyoto. It was known in Japan as Kegon, and in course of time, its teaching influenced Japanese Buddhism in general. Holistic thought always moves in whole patterns rather than analytically and its effects on Japanese society can be seen in many ways. What the subtle-minded philosophers had stated in words had long received a more concrete expression in China and Japan as the family system.

In traditional Oriental society, the family is both the basic social unit and the most important factor in individual identity. The family is on-going through time, whilst the individual is alive only briefly. Thus the individual has identity and authority only by virtue of the role he plays in the family. The most powerful person is the head of the family, hence the saying that the three things most feared by the Japanese are earthquake, typhoon and the old master. We should remember, however, that the price the master pays for his authority is a heavy onus of responsibility.

6 / EDITOR'S NOTE

In writing *Meditation Yoga*, Masahiro Oki has opened his heart in order that all may benefit from the precious truth he has gathered in the course of an unusually adventurous life. It is a completely honest presentation of his views aimed at those who have newly entered Yoga. But it is important to understand that *Meditation Yoga* expresses the philosophy of totality in its form and in content. It is not a book to be read selectively, but must be taken as a whole. From the whole emerges the spirit of *Okidō* and true meditation. This holistic spirit is a re-expression of that philosophy of totality which formerly inspired both Yoga and Buddhism. Throughout history, religion has passed through recurrent cycles of true spirituality and decline, yet religion seems to contain the power to reinstate itself. *Okidō* and *Meditation Yoga*, which are virtually synonymous, can be seen as yet another sincere attempt to restore the true spirit at a time when it has been almost lost. Because the philosophy of totality is common to all religions and ways of the spirit, *Okidō* is all-inclusive. By training men and women in the basic skills and attitudes, *Okidō* fits them to embark later upon whatever spiritual way they may choose.

Meditation Yoga is the result of the cooperation of many people. In producing this English translation I have tried, as editor, to find a balance between organizing the text for the Western mind and yet not destroying the discursive style of the traditional Oriental teacher. For example, I have expanded some passages from my knowledge of Master Oki's teaching in the interests of greater clarity but I have not attempted to alter the basic plan of the book. I am certain that *Meditation Yoga* will be of interest to those who pracitce *Okidō* and other forms of Yoga and also to students of religion and philosophy. I hope that, in spite of the perils of translation, something of the joyful, rambunctious, and disarmingly direct character of Masahiro Oki still shines through. For my part I am grateful to have had this opportunity to serve him.

September 1977   DAVID N. BRADSHAW, *Mishima*

Preface

Meditation Yoga makes you more human and led the Buddha to Enlightenment.

I have been close to religion since an early age for both my parents were devotees. My mother, a Christian, taught me to pray, help others and practice chanting. My father, a life-long Zen Buddhist, taught me the spiritual way of the martial arts and the discipline of silent sitting. His constant advice to me was this: "Develop your *Hara*, keep a positive mind and learn self-control." *Hara* is the physical and emotional center of the body, but man is also a spiritual being. He took me to many of the greatest teachers in Japan who taught me the spiritual ways of our tradition and, when I entered Junior High School, he gave me copies of the *Mumonkan* and other books which contain the most profound Buddhist wisdom. It is therefore not surprising that, even as a youngster, I was familiar with all the ideas and language of religion. Of course, I didn't have a deep understanding of many words, especially those which refer to the ultimate meaning and purpose of life. Such realization comes only from direct experience and personal attainment and I was still too young to have either. It was only later, during the course of an adventurous life filled with danger and interspersed with periods of serious illness, that I learnt to ask for divine help in my search.

Although I had studied incessantly and roamed the world seeking my spiritual teacher, I could not get any kind of deep understanding of life until I learnt both to rely upon my own efforts and, at the same time, trust the sacred power behind life. All my efforts failed to lead me to the truth until I changed my basic method. The Christ said—"Seek and ye shall find" and I had interpreted this to mean that one's own unaided efforts would eventually bring home the prize. The truth is that, although you must make maximum effort, there are no prizes to be gained but only wrong ways to be lost; no personal guarantee of success, but simple trust. It is only when you are permitted to attain the fundamental spiritual experience, which I shall call *satori*, that the profoundly religious concepts of ultimate meaning become crystal clear.

Yet, although you must accept the will of a greater power, there are certain conditions which man must fulfill by his own efforts so as to become a vessel fit to receive divine truth. This is the purpose of Meditation Yoga—*Meiso Yoga*— in all its width and depth. In my early life, I was taught Yoga and the discipline of sitting by three great teachers, Tenpu Nakamura Roshi, Ottama Daisōjō and Mahatma Gandhi. Each of my teachers explained to me that *Meiso Yoga* is the basic spiritual discipline which was common to all the great Founders of religion such as the Buddha, the Christ and the Prophet Mohammed. Some form of meditation is indispensable if you are to attain full personal development and is also the only way to learn how to relate correctly to this living universe. It was through the personal example of my teachers that I learnt that the four great principles of the spiritual life are renunciation, honesty, detachment and service. Yet it took many years before I was able to apply them fully in my own life and say—"I see and understand that it should be so."

Each person's rate of progress differs, depending upon character and strength of interest. It was not until I realized that my search for health and *satori* was a form of selfishness that I could begin to change my basic attitude. *Satori* comes only when we can put others before self, for it is giving which counts and not getting. Truth is given to us only in the course of cooperation and service; little of value can be gained by searching in isolation. It was only when I entered upon a life of service that I began to understand the real meaning of *Meiso Yoga*. Previously my mind had been attached to a variety of goals and so I was far from freedom. Detachment came when I saw that only truth is good, that truth is fact and that only what is necessary is of real value. Yoga is the search for truth and *Meiso Yoga* is the unification of four great principles. These are the integration of the body through the breath, the concentration of the mind through Zen discipline, the heart of worship and the experience of *satori*. Although I had strenuously practiced the first two, I could not attain *satori* because I lacked the heart of worship. A mind which imposes conditions upon our actions is a barrier to spiritual progress but worship gradually corrects this habit. I also learnt that we must learn to live entirely in the present and that, when we do, our everyday, mundane life becomes an exciting theater of spiritual training. The way of life which is based upon this realization is *Meiso Yoga*. At first I had completely misunderstood meditation, thinking that it is just sitting practice. In fact it is the deliberate creation, step by step, of a unified body and mind which becomes our precious instrument for understanding truth and coming to freedom. In *Meiso Yoga* we learn to use every experience to develop ourselves for the good of all and not merely for self. Zen discipline gives not only physical stability, but also creates a balance between tension and relaxation. The worshipful mind likewise brings balance between the utmost mental effort and complete tranquility. *Satori* means being able to accept, bear and creatively use the pain of life while living only in the present and being totally in the service of others. When these three are established and work as one, you can know reality as it is, understand everything precisely and feel correctly. By being able to appreciate the true worth of all beings, including yourself, you can see the Sacred everywhere. Then the mind of real appreciation and the heart of worship arise spontaneously and this is Enlightenment.

    This state in which you are manifesting your full value and ability is called *Kensho*. When such a mind is turned inwards you know yourself and when it is turned outwards to others it is called *satori*. To live only in the present and to serve others with true Buddhist detachment is called *Hoetsu* and it can arise only from a profound realization of the Sacred. In the *Kensho* condition man has become divine so that *Meiso Yoga* not only develops personality and humanity but also leads to sainthood. Alternatively, we can say that it helps us to recover our original nature to which we now add experience and understanding. Balance gives us detachment and the ability to communicate with others at the deepest. *Meiso Yoga* leads to balance and also provides both a philosophy and a religion.

The real joy of life appears when we can unify nature and culture, wealth and poverty, movement and stillness, attachment and detachment. Unfortunately, we all have a long way to go in this direction and it is here that *Meiso Yoga* can serve both the individual and society. Yoga is neither a sect nor an ideology but a practical training of mind and body. Broadly speaking, it has three main outcomes: it makes you more aware of your natural wisdom, or *Bussho*; it strengthens the body's ability to recover from illness or injury; it teaches us how to cooperate with others. Because *Meiso Yoga* teaches truth through mind and body rather than theory, it brings about deep changes of attitude. People typically become more affirmative, gain balance and detachment, and are less inclined to compete, to avoid what is unpleasant and to reject other's opinions out of hand. The entire thrust of your life is to devote total attention to every action and, at the same time, to trust in the power of the Sacred.

Meiso Yoga thus blends the two states of tension and relaxation. Life always seeks to restore balance and the ideal state is that in which static force and dynamic power are in harmony. In this state, the deepest relaxation is found within the highest tension and this forms the basis for the new life of service and cooperation. *Meiso Yoga* is very far from being just a technique for gaining the limited goals of concentration, emptiness, calmness or ecstasy but seeks to integrate the life of all beings into a harmonious whole. Those religions which recognize the presence of the Sacred in all things also assist wholeness by creating a situation in which self and others can be most secure. This philosophy of life is neither old nor new, but eternal, neither Oriental nor Occidental but rooted in *satori*, for when *satori* forms the basis of thought, all differences vanish and evil is neutralized.

I dedicate this book to all who seek the Way. It is a guide for those who wish to enter the Way of Yoga which they will find to be the most reasonable and natural route to *satori*. It is my intention to publish a second volume later which will deal with the more advanced stages of the spiritual path.

Contents

Editor's Note 5
Preface 7

Chapter 1   WHAT IS YOGA?   13

    1. Yogic Meditation   13
    2. Yoga is Both Physical and Spiritual   18
    3. The Origin of Yoga   22
    4. The Philosophy of Yoga   28
    5. The God of Yoga   34

Chapter 2   BASIC TRAINING   39

    1. The Eight Stages of Yoga   39
    2. The First Stage   43
    3. Niyama, The Second Stage   45
    4. The Third Stage: Asanas and Dōzen   48
    5. The Fourth and Fifth Stages: Diet and Breath Control   59

Chapter 3   MEDITATION   81

    1. The Width and Depth of Yogic Meditation   81
    2. The Real Meaning of Unification and Detachment   86
    3. Dharana: The Sixth Stage   90
    4. The Seventh Stage   103
    5. Satori: The Eighth and Highest Stage   120

Chapter 4   PERSONAL EXPERIENCES   127

    1. Meiso Yoga in the Dōjō   127
    2. The Sacred in Gaol—The Teaching of Hoseini-shi   137
    3. The Uses of Fear in Esoteric Religious Systems   149

Glossary 161
List of Okidō Address 167
Index 169

Chapter 1 What Is Yoga?

1. Yogic Meditation

When most people think about meditation, they visualize pious souls deeply absorbed in prayer or gray bearded philosophers dreaming about ideas. In the West, Pascal's view of meditation reinforces these images, for he described it as deep, tranquil thought. Yet, in Yoga and Buddhism as well as in Oriental philosophy in general, meditation has a very different and far more precise connotation. Strangely enough, in the early period of Christianity and Islam, meditation did not mean just quiet pondering, for it also involved certain rigorous preparations. In fact all the religions of ancient times taught very specific procedures in relation to entering upon periods of meditation. For example, it is clear from the sacred writings of their religions that the Buddha, the Christ and the Prophet Mohammed each practiced prayer and fasting before withdrawing to some isolated place to meditate.

These procedures, or spiritual disciplines, are common to all religions because they mirror the realities of human nature and the hardships of the search for the supreme way of life. This universal wisdom, or perennial philosophy, has been continuously handed down by the many groups which have, at all times, sought the truth. It is simply the spiritual common sense that leads most directly to a higher level of consciousness. If the reader actually practices Yogic meditation, he will soon see that these basic disciplines are vital in order to integrate mind and body. Only then can he pass onwards to that experience of oneness with reality which is called *satori*. These preparations establish the right physical and mental posture for effective meditation. This can be described as follows:

Physical 1. A stabilized posture which is, in fact, the natural

		body.
	2.	Balanced breath and the practice of right diet.
Mental	1.	Original mind, detached, purified, strengthened and active.
	2.	The mind of faith arising from a developed *Hara* center.

All these factors will be more fully described later.

Yoga began at least six thousand years ago and has continuously been enriched by the wisdom accumulating from humanity's struggle for survival. But such practices as right posture, correct breathing and sound diet have a wider relevance, for they can be seen as the factors necessary for maintaining the integrity of the Life-Force, health, society and even the cosmic laws. Out of these practices is generated the state of mind necessary for meditation as well as the possibility of harmonious relationships and cooperation between all living beings. In other words, Yoga took the best of the scientific endeavors of every age and combined this knowledge with the science of life. It embraces the spiritual disciplines as well as those techniques of healing which human beings need to bring them more closely in touch with the body and mind.

Because of this wide base, Yoga does not conflict with modern medical science or with psychology but actually explains certain contradictions and gaps in modern knowledge. As the essence of so much precious human experience, Yoga goes beyond the limits of present understanding and teaches, for example, the way to transcendental consciousness. The basic characteristic of Yoga is its use of meditation, for by utilizing this discipline, the mind and body are purified and adjusted and personality is heightened. By means of a gradual process, Yoga enables everyone to move towards that state of developed consciousness which is oneness with the Sacred. The first step is to harmonize, purify and strengthen both body and mind. It is a path which is open to all and rewards all who tread it.

Modern civilization has developed during the last five hundred years as a direct result of the discoveries of science. By contrast, Yoga has developed, over a far longer period, the skills of living in tune with nature. The words "nature" and "natural" used in connection with Yoga do not mean "primitive," but rather the ability to be perfectly adjusted to all situations including the relatively new and extreme situation called modern life.

The most rational way of seeing the interrelations with exist between man and nature is that of Yoga. Yet, we should ask why Yoga alone has been able to adopt only the best features of other religions and philosophies and how it has managed to remain free from prejudice, narrow-mindedness and conflict? Since its earliest beginnings, Yoga has been generated by self-governing groups of free thinkers who have rejected any fixed ideology. Only that which a man could try and test for himself has been accepted as the truth and, in ancient times, Yogins were actually called *Samon*, which means free-thinkers who set up no school and adhered to no set forms of activity. Their sole aim was to follow the spiritual path and the practice which was, and is, appropriate to this is meditation.

To know the relationship between oneself and the cosmos in the most profound sense is both meditation and the result of meditation. Thus there is no goal in meditation except goallessness. The primary attitude of Yoga is not that of scholarly achievement; it is far more holistic. It is to steadily refine the individual personality according to the ideal of Enlightenment, which is oneness with the Sacred. Yoga conducts us along this path by giving us a step by step experience of ourselves beginning at the physical level. Meditation is therefore not simply a mental discipline, but one which integrates mind and body, bringing the individual into a state of harmony with the universe.

What is the posture that we associate with thinking? Rodin's famous sculpture "the Thinker" springs immediately to mind, yet the posture of the masterpiece and its entire expression are quite different from what I associate with meditation. In fact for me, Rodin's creation symbolizes suffering and reflects what everyone experiences, the pain and suffering of the human condition. There are many sculptures of the Buddha in meditation and most of them show a stable, upright posture in which the spine is extended and held straight. It is very rare, however, to find one which completely represents the posture necessary for meditation. For example, the

Japanese Miroku, the Buddha of the future, represents the body leaning slightly forward and the face lit by an expression of warmth and affection. It conveys perfectly the spirit of Indian Yogic meditation.

I have practiced many forms of meditation in Japan, Tibet, China, India, Arabia and the Middle East. All of them called their practice "meditation" but the character and effect of each was different. *Meiso Yoga*—the meditation of Okidō—brings together three basic elements: Zen discipline for the development of *Hara*, the joy and rapture of Buddhist insight meditation, and the quality of worship found in Sufi and Christian meditation. The differences between the various forms of meditation arose from the different character of each religion and the circumstances attending its development. Indian meditation chiefly emphasizes relaxation whilst Japanese meditation, especially in Rinzai Zen, finds peace in the highest tension. Islamic and Christian meditation is a third factor, the offering of the self to the Sacred through worship. Although the quality and rationale of the meditation is different in each case, the underlying principle is the same. Therefore the three can be unified according to the principle of *Sanmitsu*, the harmony of three. It is when we look only at the techniques employed in reflective meditation, or pondering, concentration practice, or detachment and so on, that we think there are different kinds of meditation. All these are unified in the true meditation of *Meiso Yoga*.

In Japanese, the word "Meiso," means meditation. This symbol carries a wide range of meaning since it conveys the concept of "all" and includes the ideas of the past, present and future, whether viewed as real or abstract categories. In fact "mei" does not originate at the conceptual level but arises from deeper layers of consciousness. If I call this the realm of no-thought it should not be confused with vacuity or absent mindedness. Rather it is a state of consciousness which is empty of contingent contents—thoughts about this and that—and so it is empty of limitation, being universal. Because it is characterized by emptiness it is free to know the reality of all things by directly uniting with them. *Satori* is thus a state in which mind and body are functioning as one and the subject unites with the object. Objects are apperceived directly, clearly and peacefully, yet without any attachment.

Meditation is a training in introspection—listening to the inner voices. This is the voice of life which speaks *Hannya*, the wisdom of nature. Human wisdom consists in two things: the disposition to regain and maintain the power of self-healing and *bussho*, the faculty of real understanding. Only when we learn to follow the promptings of *Hannya* can we gain real health and *satori*. *Satori* produces your own profound understanding of life and truth—which *is* your inner being. Now we can see that Yogic meditation is a life-science which respects scientific knowledge but leads us to deeper wisdom.

Yoga is both the way of health and the way of self-discovery. In Yoga we are guided by the inner teacher, the voice of life. The Latin word for meditation means deep inner reflection but true meditation does not at all mean quiet pondering. It is far more dynamic and means making the mind and body one—in the peacefulness of *satori* we go far beyond thought. Zen training, especially, has been the subject of much scientific research, but I do not think that such disciplines as physiology or psychology in their present forms can fully grasp the real meaning and effects of meditation. *Meiso Yoga* combines the stability of body and mind as taught in Zen, the joy of *satori*, and the attitude of worship. But since science today is chiefly concerned with the physiological effects resulting from mental stimuli, it can measure only the first of these three.

To unify the mind and body it is necessary to balance the influence of the cortex—the self-conscious part of the brain—with the influence of the *Hara*—the center of the autonomic nervous system which is responsible for life-maintenance. Of course it is important to know the direct physical and mental effects of Zen meditation and to see how it can enhance physical functioning, clear the mind and establish concentration. But this approach lacks the conceptual framework and the practical means to estimate the effect of the religious mind. At the present time, the scientific measurement of faith is impossible, yet faith is a vital factor for the attainment of *satori*.

2. Yoga Is Both Physical and Spiritual

Yoga is an age old method for recovering and developing the individuality of human beings which was long kept secret. There are, today, many misunderstandings about Yoga, especially concerning its use of *asanas* which bend the body into extreme postures. Those who see these curious contortions, sometimes suppose that this is the whole of Yoga, but this is not the case. We can say the same about meditation methods and, because Indian Yoga has contributed a great deal to this general confusion, I believe that Indian Yoga is no longer true Yoga. As a basic reference point I say that Yoga is that which was practiced by the Buddha and, later, by Mahatma Gandhi.

As I have already said, Yoga is never extreme or unnatural, but is actually the most reasonable way of conducting individual and social life. Yoga is the way of discovering how to live best and to create the ideal society. Japan has had long experience of Yoga and has absorbed something of its true spirit into her culture since Yoga has deeply influenced the religious teachings which have been transmitted here. The main purpose of this book is to try to give the reader a feeling for the spirit of true Yoga and not to teach sectarian doctrine or training methods.

The Buddha is respected by people throughout the world and especially in Japan, for he was a man who gained full and perfect Enlightenment through Yoga. It is quite evident that his teaching was Yoga reinterpreted and raised to the level of religion. But most of the present day Buddhist sects in Japan have developed from one or other of the Sutras and so they have lost the philosophy of totality which is characteristic of true Yoga. Modern Buddhism seems to have lost its vitality and no longer leads the people along the real path to Enlightenment. Although you may think it is strange to say that Buddhism is Yoga, this is only because people fail to see the Yogic ideal embodied in the original Buddhist teaching on account of the confusion caused by present day sectarian presentations. In India, the word "yoga" is commonplace, but its true reference is to a practical training method leading to unification, stability and self-control. This practical reference is of far greater importance than any theoretical component, which is almost non-existent. Consequently, Yoga can only be comprehended through practice and not simply through conceptual study. It is strange that some people should think they can grasp Yoga in an academic way and this is symptomatic of the analytical mode of Western thought which tends to mistake the brain for the total human organism. There is a saying in the Orient—"Those who read the Analects of Confucius many times do not understand Confucius." The point is that the Analects are intended to be put into practice in your daily life and not merely cogitated upon. We can say the same thing for Yoga, for a person who practices only the *asanas* and *pranayama* will never really understand Yoga because he does not live a totally Yogic life-style.

For this reason, you cannot award grades in Yoga, for how can you judge a person's total progress in life? The Martial Arts of Japan used to be spiritual disciplines but today there is much commercialism based on the sale of *dan* grades. There are relatively few teachings like Okidō, which aim only at purity and truth. Even those who have lived and practiced in the Dōjō for many years have no rank or status and all members, including myself, are equally privileged. Thus we have no managers, or leaders but only those who serve. Our common aim is to strive for self-control, true humanity and Enlightenment whilst serving others in a spirit of love. We aim at the Bodhisattva ideal of mental purification and the resuscitation of the natural recovery powers of the body. The Okidō Dōjōs are the only centers in the world today which fully embody these principles in a practical life-style.

In modern times it has been largely forgotten that practical self-training is man's most noble estate. Like all modern people, the Japanese have also changed for the worst and now pay attention only to what can be understood easily and instantly. This is the basic reason for the maladies of modern society. We can never experience the full joy of life without practical spiritual training to cultivate ourselves and attain perfect balance. Because we have been born at a time when an unnatural life-style prevails, we need Yoga training more than ever before to help us recover our real nature. We especially need to acquire adaptability and stamina and the way is Yoga. Yoga's basic method is the three-fold one of spiritual training, physical training and the systematic application of the knowledge we gain to our daily lives. I will explain this method in greater detail later, but the harmonious combination of these three phases is the most reasonable way of life and the true practice of *Meiso Yoga*.

At first I rejected the present title of this book because I thought people would mistake it for yet another book about Indian Yoga or modern Buddhism. I have experienced many different kinds of meditation but I finally derived the most inspiration from Yoga and so developed *Meiso Yoga* as the best way to help people to discover their original nature. At first I had wanted to call the book *The Meditation of the Buddha*, but I realized that people would associate this also with modern Buddhism. I then considered *A Method of Meditation Practice*, but this has no reference to Yoga. Finally I chose *Meditation Yoga: The Meiso Yoga of Okidō* because of my debt to Yoga for helping me to understand that although there are many different forms of meditation, the aim of all is the same. Although different words are used in the different religions, the common aim is Enlightenment, which is *satori* seen in its aspect of religious ecstasy. In this book I want to explain the path to Enlightenment stage by stage so that everyone can understand clearly and practice. In the second volume, which I intend to write soon, I will give an objective account of Enlightenment, of the religious mind, and of the importance of *Hara* for the physical and spiritual development of human beings.

Even though it is impossible to write a detailed history of Yoga, it is necessary to know something of Yoga's background in order to see how it acquired its present form. Religious teachers were plentiful in ancient India and we know that each one tended to emphasize one aspect of discipline. Some taught the way of ascetic self-control whilst others taught methods of correcting physical distortions. Some taught strengthening exercises and other taught the purification of body and mind, the raising of consciousness, ways of stabilization or of harmony. What all of them shared was a preoccupation with the end result and an emphasis on practice.

For these reasons, there are almost no written texts about their teachings, yet the Indian memory is such that all this knowledge was preserved and eventually brought together to form what we now know as Yoga. The *Samkhya* teaching gave Yoga a philosophical framework and *Vedanta* later added idealism and logic. But as Indian civilization developed, Yoga became more and more comprehensive and sophisticated, serving as an education system, a technology and a spiritual training. Yoga cared for the health of body and mind, advanced the study of psychic phenomena and provided a means of cultivating supernormal powers. In fine, Yoga became an encyclopedic method according to which man's entire life is a training ground for seeking the truth.

It is said that there are seventy-two different formulations of the Yogic way and that all of them lead to Enlightenment. These ways are not identical with specific religious sects but represent individual spirituals paths. I have chosen one of these ways as a means of structuring this book: it is the Yoga of eight stages which was systematized by *Patanjali*. This is sometimes called *Astanga Yoga* or *Raja Yoga*. The reason for my choice is that the eight stages give a clear, logical structure and aid the progressive development of understanding.

Those who teach *Hatha Yoga* have, often unwittingly, caused misconceptions about the true nature of Yoga, yet the fact is that *Hatha Yoga* is the most widely taught today. In many cases it is presented as being purely physical, although it was not so originally. Most authorities agree, however, that *Raja Yoga* is the mainstream of spiritual Yoga despite the fact that it also contains the *asanas*, rules of diet, and *pranayama* for the purification of body, mind and spirit. In fact *Hatha Yoga* was derived from *Raja Yoga* by teachers who placed most emphasis on physical exercise and it is today regarded by many people as being a preparation for *Raja Yoga*. But those who claim that either of these is real Yoga, or even both together, do not know Yoga. Real Yoga must embrace these two as well as *Jnana*, *Bhakti* and *Karma Yoga* which are the Yogas of philosophy, worship and service, respectively.

The background to *Raja Yoga* is *Samkhya*, whilst *Jnana* and

Bhakti are linked to *Vedanta* even though these two forms of Yoga seem very different. Whilst *Jnana* in its *Raja* and *Hatha Yoga* forms was non-theistic, *Bhakti Yoga* was essentially the Yoga of devotion and worship. For the *Bhakti* Yogin, everything he sees is God and therefore sacred and at first I could not understand how two such very different things could both be Yoga. I felt that it was very much easier to seek the truth by means of one clear-cut teaching. There is always conflict, antagonism and useless vituperation in religion because of conflicting doctrines and this serves only to disrupt the social structure and cause violence. But until I realized the true nature of Yoga I was also influenced by this partisan attitude which adopts an extreme position and seeks to convert or destroy all who are in opposition. I felt that a firm and resolute stance in philosophy and religion was essential for a man of genuine faith. Yoga opened my mind to the truth that such a view is narrow, biased and divisive in its effects. Mahatma Gandhi influenced me deeply by his deep faith and genuinely universal love. I hope that subsequent chapters of this book will help the reader to understand that Yoga is a religion which bridges East and West and combines all that is best in philosophy, religion and science. In the modern world, Yoga is actually the only teaching which is potentially a universal religion and way of salvation. Because it combines every viewpoint and every method, only Yoga can help us to attain our full stature as persons, and holiness, without denying others the right to live in their own way. I sincerely hope that the reader will clearly grasp this key point.

3. The Origin of Yoga

We do not know for certain when Yoga began, but it was at least six thousand years ago. The people of the northern Indian city-state, *Mohenjo Dharo,* had statues of a God who is shown seated in the Yogic "lotus" position. *Mohenjo Dharo* was located in what is now Pakistan, on the estuary of the River Indus and it was an agrarian society of pre-Aryan people. I have visited the site of this once great city on two occasions, but it is not clear to what extent Yoga was developed in those ancient times. The work of the archaeologists does establish, however, that Yoga was known and practiced before the Aryan invasions.

The Aryan religion of Brahmanism incorporated elaborate rituals of sacrifice and was based on the ancient texts called the *Vedas*. We know that Brahmanism was introduced by the Aryans because the script used in the *Vedas* is quite different from that used by the indigenous *Dravidian* people of *Mohenjo Dharo* and the Indus valley. In spite of its complex ceremonies, Brahmanism can be clearly understood in its basic principles. The word "Veda" means "knowledge" and the first Vedas were brought to India between 2000 B.C. and 1500 B.C. By that time the civilization of the Indus valley was already in decline and *Mohenjo Dharo* retained only a little of its former splendor. Brahmanism has many Gods which it absorbed from Iran and the Indus valley area, but the chief trinity is *Siva, Vishnu* and *Brahma*. *Brahman* is not a God, but the mysterious and all-pervading power behind the universe. The early *Vedas* contain no mention of Yoga but only the name and idea of *Brahman* and the names of the subordinate Gods. Long before the time of the Christ, we find in India these two main streams: the religion of the Aryans and the religion of the *Samon* of the Indus valley. *Samon* means "freedom" and their religion did contain aspects of Yoga, so that it seems safe to say that the *Samon* were early Yogins. The word "Brahman" has the connotation of "intellectual"—it was a religion which placed little emphasis on practice, consisting mainly of theology, hymns and ritual. At the end of the Rig Veda, which was the earliest Veda, we encounter the word *"tapas"* for the first time. *Tapas* means "inner fire" or spiritual power and some scholars claim that this indicates a knowledge of Yoga. I do not agree with them, however, because although Yoga develops *tapas*, it does so in the opposite way to Brahmanism. The *tapas* of the Vedas is developed through hard, ascetic discipline, but Yoga works through peace, stability and relaxation of body and mind. Even when I was fully engaged in Yoga training, I enjoyed the practice and experienced no inner resistance such as would be the natural reaction to asceticism.

Vedas

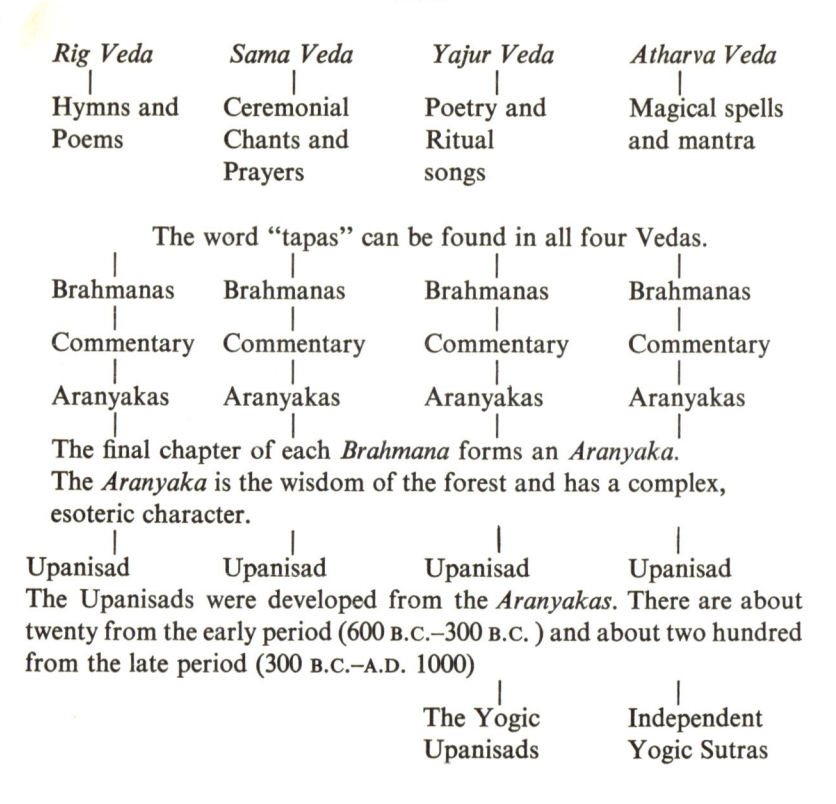

Rig Veda	Sama Veda	Yajur Veda	Atharva Veda
Hymns and Poems	Ceremonial Chants and Prayers	Poetry and Ritual songs	Magical spells and mantra

The word "tapas" can be found in all four Vedas.

Brahmanas	Brahmanas	Brahmanas	Brahmanas
Commentary	Commentary	Commentary	Commentary
Aranyakas	Aranyakas	Aranyakas	Aranyakas

The final chapter of each *Brahmana* forms an *Aranyaka*. The *Aranyaka* is the wisdom of the forest and has a complex, esoteric character.

| Upanisad | Upanisad | Upanisad | Upanisad |

The Upanisads were developed from the *Aranyakas*. There are about twenty from the early period (600 B.C.–300 B.C.) and about two hundred from the late period (300 B.C.–A.D. 1000)

| | The Yogic Upanisads | Independent Yogic Sutras |

The Brahmanistic religion is thus theologically orientated, ritualistic, and included the practice of ingesting an hallucinogenic drug called *soma* which gave ecstatic experiences. Yoga is quite different since it aims at stability and peace and possesses an entirely different character to the Aryan religion. Brahmanism is concerned with vivid, exciting experience and the fire of *tapas*. Yoga and its illustrious child, Buddhism, is the religion of silence and peace. *Nirvana* is often described as "cooling," or "blowing out the flame of desire." Nevertheless, this clear distinction between Brahmanism and Yoga did not persist in later times in India, for there grew up a Brahmanistic Yoga. Only in Buddhism do we find the true principles of Yoga continuing, according to which silent meditation must be balanced by dynamic action. When the Yin and Yang forces of mind and body are developed to the utmost and unified, the mind of *Mu*, or emptiness is the result. *Mu* mind goes far beyond anything that can be attained merely by concentration and this was first discovered by the Buddha. In later times it has been reconfirmed and demonstrated by Mahatma Gandhi.

Because Yoga combines all paths and, even though it may sometimes appear to contradict itself, it is actually the way of balance for all mankind. The Yogic path is free and uninhibited and, since its fundamental practice is meditation, we can say that Yoga is meditation. The perfect meditation practiced by the Buddha, the Christ, the Prophet Mohammed and Mahatma Gandhi is *Meiso Yoga*. Western people are often attracted to Buddhism because it is a natural religion of calmness which emphasizes the middle way of moderation. Indeed Buddhism has a deep logic which goes beyond normal rationality and this is also found in the Upanisads. There is some evidence that there was mutual influence between the Upanisads and Buddhism, for both were reactions to Brahmanism which became degenerate and declined in spiritual power.

The word "Upanisad" means "to sit near" and we can imagine the teacher and the student sitting face to face and the teacher expounding the secret lore of the sacred texts.

The old Upanisads, which were written between 600 B.C. and 300 B.C. were contemporary with both the Buddha and Mahavira, the founder of Jainism, who were both actively teaching at that time. The technology of Indian civilization had reached the stage of the development of iron and its use in the manufacture of implements and weapons. Religion, too, was correspondingly well developed and had already given rise to a sophisticated philosophy. Although the authors of the Upanisads were separated by both time and distance, their writings present a unified picture of the stages of man's spiritual development in terms of the Indian world view. The Upanisads are the philosophy of Brahmanism and deal with its ultimate goal—the union of the individual life with the life of the cosmos. One of the oldest Upanisads, the *Taittiriya*, refers directly to Yoga when it says—"Yoga is the union of Atman and Brahman and Yoga is strength." Some of the earlier Upanisads explain Yoga in some detail, but mention only six stages. In the later Upanisads we find an early form of *Raja Yoga*, a Yoga of eight stages. These are as follows:

1. *Yama*   The universal moral laws.
2. *Niyama*   Personal moral rules of conduct.
3. *Asana*   Yogic postures.
4. *Pranayama*   Acquiring and controlling *prana*, or energy, by means of the breath.
5. *Pratyahara* The withdrawal of the senses from the outer environment.
6. *Dharana*   Concentration.
7. *Dhyana*   Meditation.
8. *Samadhi*   Enlightenment.

Even at the time of the Buddha, there was a systematic Yoga which had entered Brahmanism from outside. This happened at a time of conflict between the *Brahmins*, or priests and the *Ksatreyas*, or warriors. Social forms were changing as a result of the development of iron and the warriors had become immensely more powerful with the manufacture of iron weapons. In consequence of this and the general decline of Brahmanism, they now sought freedom from the traditional domination of the priests. The Buddha came from the *Shakya* tribe and Mahavira from the *Natas* and both were of aristocratic, warrior blood. What was new in the religions which they inspired was the renunciation of worldly power, for neither of them wished to become an important priest or king. They were *Samon*, men who sought freedom and truth, and they were protected at this time by the warriors of the Magadan kingdom which is now the modern state of Bihar. Their sole interest was to engage in the practical aspects of man's search for spiritual truth for the benefit of others. In modern times, the greatest exponent of this path was Mahatma Gandhi.

There is a close resemblance between the Upanisads and some of the Sutras of Jainism and Buddhism. The style of all three is rational and all extol practice, for Yoga formed the core of the reaction against Brahmanism. Brahmanism also adopted Yoga at a later time and this helped it to regain its vitality. Indeed, there was continuous interaction between all these groups so that we find aspects of Brahmanism included in the *Upanisads* even though it is fundamentally opposed to Yoga. A Yogic amalgam of Indian religion thus began to develop about 300 B.C. and attained its zenith when the Buddhist Emperor Asoka (272 B.C.–232 B.C.) came to power and unified India. Although Asoka extended full freedom to all religions, Brahmanism declined seriously during his reign, for it was no longer the state religion and could not depend upon state finance. But under subsequent non-Buddhist Emperors, Brahmanism again returned to a position of power and prestige and Buddhism was eventually exiled from the land of its birth. Jainism too contracted, continuing only as the religion of a small, but influential group, whilst Yoga in its independent form survived only amongst small groups who practiced meditation and who were never fully integrated into regular society.

Yoga, as the only religion without a Founder, lays great stress on self-reliance, independence and flexibility and this is why it has managed to avoid absorption by other religions. Yoga is essentially practice, so it has not given rise to a sacred literature on which could be built any kind of orthodoxy. At the present time, Yoga exists chiefly as the fundamental discipline at the heart of all religions. It was from Mahatma ("great soul") Gandhi, that I learnt the profound truth of Yoga as well as much about religion, meditation, fasting and life.

So Yoga, the religious discipline of the *Samon*, penetrated deeply into Brahmanism and permanently influenced its way of thought. At the same time, the warrior caste protected Yoga and unified India. Although the Brahmin priests at first resisted Yoga, the intelligent people of the time accepted it as the basis for a spiritual regeneration. Later, the Brahmins, too, were obliged to modify their basically theoretical orientation by incorporating the experiential attitude of Yoga along with the indigenous wisdom of India which Yoga preserved. Yoga, as the wisdom of life, is the essence of the cumulative experience of many great minds, yet even Yoga develops specific cultural forms. So when you take up Yoga, you should consider your own environment and personality. Recognizing this, Okidō is taught differently within each culture. For example, the Yogins of ancient India alternated between meditating in their forest Ashrams during the rainy season and wandering among the villages at other times. This life-style is still followed by many in India today. Even though Indian society still recognizes and accepts the vocation of the wandering priest-Yogin, it is obvious that Yoga must take different forms in modern industrialized societies.

The Brahmanistic religion was at first disdainful of the indigenous wisdom of India, but after the 6th Century B.C. the situation rapidly changed. From then onwards, Yogic concepts appeared, not only in the *Upanisads*, but also in the Brahmanistic epic scripture, the *Mahabharata*. Indeed, the *Bhagavad Gita*, which is part of the *Mahabharata*, contains the very heart of Yoga. So, too, the teaching of the Buddha can be seen as a sophisticated development of integral Yoga to which has been added something precious and unique. So Yoga is today found in Hinduism—the name given to amalgum of Brahmanism and Yoga—in Buddhism and in Jainism. Yoga has contributed the ideal of self-renunciation and service to these religions, as exemplified in the lives of the Buddha and Mahatma Gandhi, as well as a developed and refined spiritual ascesis. Yet, in the entire history of the human race, the Buddha alone has taken Yoga to its fullest and final conclusion.

4. The Philosophy of Yoga

In the Upanisads, Yoga became much more philosophical and, consequently, had a great deal in common with 'Buddhistic ways of thought and practice. Some Brahmanistic writings too were influenced by Yoga, as for example, the *Katha Upanisad*, which dates from about the 6th Century B.C. Here we find a simile used to explain Yoga as the "yoking" of body and mind, much as two horses are yoked together to draw a chariot. Some time later, the *Kataka Upanisad* develops this same simile as follows: "The body is the vehicle, the senses are the horses, the whip is consciousness, the driver is rationality, but the owner of the coach is the Atman, or self, who travels inside." This simile seems very apt because the fundamental meaning of Yoga is to control the body and mind through the activity of consciousness.

In the *Svetasvatara Upanisad*, the central practice of Yoga is explained as follows: "Stretch the spine and neck upwards, calm the mind, control the senses and let consciousness ride on the ship of Aum to cross over the ocean of fear." Another significant sentence from the same *Upanisad* is as follows: "The mind is like a dusty mirror which, if cleaned, regains the ability to reflect clearly." If we can pass beyond regret and unify the mind, we can attain to *satori*. It would help the reader if he could keep these two quotations in mind when reading *Meiso Yoga*.

By about 2nd Century B. C., Brahmanism had given rise to six schools of philosophy. These were:

1. *Mimasa* — The philosophy of the Vedic rituals.
2. *Vedanta* — The philosophy of the unification of Brahman and Atman. Vedanta later became a very influential school.
3. *Samkhya* — An atheistic system based on analysis which accounts for the world in terms of two fundamental principles which interact with each other. These are *Purusa*, or spirit, and *Prakrti*, matter or nature.
4. *Yoga* — Discipline through which we seek to become unconditioned and so attain salvation. The more we can free ourselves from selfishness the nearer we shall be to the Divine. Yoga is the philosophy of gradual self-improvement and, although it was near to *Samkhya* in some respects, it was neither atheistic nor did it have its own iconog-

5. *Vaisesika* raphy.
This school of philosophy maintained the real existence of the following:
   a) Essence in the sense of soul, or substance.
   b) Quality.
   c) Movement.
   d) Immutability—nothing can be transmuted into another form.
   e) Individuality.
   f) Immanence—the Sacred is present in all things.
6. *Nyaya* This school paid special attention to the laws of logic and was similar in some ways to the Vaisesika.

From about the time when the old *Upanisads* were transcribed, Yoga and *Samkhya* developed together and *Samkhya* provided Yoga with a developed philosophy. When we speak of *Samkhya*, we usually mean an atheistic dualism, but we should note that *Samkhya Yoga* was not atheistic. The word "*Samkhya*" means "to count": life should be viewed rationally and all events should be analyzed in terms of cause and effect. Through this process of logical analysis, we progressively gain detachment and free ourselves from the entanglements of nature so that we can return to the spirit, which is our true self. Although *Samkhya* is chiefly known in its Yogic form, the *Kapila* people developed an independent *Samkhya* school about the 4th or 5th Century B.C. What was common to both *Samkhya* and *Samkhya Yoga* was the method of calm, rational analysis, but whilst *Samkhya Yoga* sought to reunite the soul with the greater life of the cosmos, personified as *Ishvara, Samkhya* aimed only to enable the self to regain awareness of itself as the principle of consciousness. This difference is important and colors the entire fabric of *Samkhya Yoga* philosophy since it admits the powerful factor of faith.

The Yoga Sutra of *Patanjali* tells us about the Yoga that had developed in ancient times and provides a sort of text book of the spiritual life. It tells us about *Raja Yoga*, the Yoga of the mind, as well as *Hatha Yoga*, the Yoga of the body. *Patanjali* puts into a systematic form all the wisdom of the Yogic tradition and it is clear that he must have been a great Yogin himself. In present day Yoga systems there are almost always eight stages, or steps, mentioned and this classification is derived from the Yoga Sutra of *Patanjali*. However, in Okidō, ten stages are recognized. Now, although the Yoga Sutra is immensely valuable we should not presume that all development of Yoga ceased after *Patanjali*'s time! Yoga is seeking the way through personal experience. It is the religion of movement and life and we should not allow it to lose its characteristic freedom by becoming tied to any one person's views. In the sense that what we are not yet ready to understand is hidden from us, Yoga is an esoteric religion. Such religion has little use for theory or the written word.

In later times, Yoga was taught from many different angles so that the tradition is that there are seventy-two "gates" or "paths" to *satori*. The aim of Okidō is to give the basic training and establish the basic attitudes which are necessary to enter any of these gates. When we can realize through our own experience that, not only is the preparation the same, but that all paths lead to the same destination, then we will deeply feel the unity of life. Work and leisure should be indistinguishable, for every situation becomes a teacher. The Buddhist ideal of the *Bosatsu*, or *Bodhisattva*, is associated with this way of practice, which was derived from Yoga. In earlier years I had sought to realize the truth through isolated meditation but all my efforts were in vain. It was only when I recognized that all phases of life are equally valuable opportunities for self-improvement and that the sole purpose of life is to find the Way, that I experienced *satori* and knew the truth of Emptiness.

The seventy-two gates to *satori* can be classified as follows:

1. *Jnana Yoga*   The Yoga of philosophy which reached its greatest development with the Buddhist teacher Nagajuna.
2. *Bhakti Yoga*   The purification of mind and body through faith as in the Lotus sects and Jodo Shin-

3. *Raja Yoga* shu.
Controlling the fluctuations of the mind as in Zen.
4. *Hatha Yoga* The discipline of physical and mental control like the *Sennin* of the mountains.
5. *Kriya Yoga* The Yoga of techniques for purifying mind and body.
6. *Mantra Yoga* The Yoga of chanting and worship—Shingon-shu.
7. *Karma Yoga* The Yoga of service to others.

The seventy-two gates, here condensed into seven groups, are methods of practice, not religious schools or sects. They are all embodied in Okidō, which not only teaches the basic preparation, but also encourages students to discover their own individual way. There is much overlapping of the seven groups, of course, but the basic emphasis of each gate is different. For example, we cannot really separate *asanas* and breathing, or *Bhakti* and *Mantra Yoga*.

Yoga begins when you make the conscious decision to improve yourself, then you can choose your Way and gradually, through practice, reach successively more advanced stages. Finally, we can grasp the meaning of our lives, know our true self, and become, for the first time, fully human. For such reasons, no-one can tell another which is the best way; you must discover your own way by yourself. In Okidō, we make a sincere attempt to help those who have completed their basic training to discover this unique path. Yoga seeks to heighten personality and bring out true individuality, so everyone may become his own Savior.

The first objective is to train yourself to cooperate harmoniously with others at the highest level. *Satori* means seeing no difference between self and others and this is the mind of Yoga. According to the simile of the coach and horses, Yoga teaches us how to strengthen the vehicle which carries us through life by our own efforts. We should not permit the vehicle to be dragged in any random direction by the horses of sense-pleasure, but should consciously decide where we wish to go. If we give attention to details and try to keep a flexible

The Philosophy of Yoga / 33

mind we can enjoy the rhythm of the vehicle as it travels on its way. When he was young, Wolfgang Mozart composed and played many lovely pieces of music whilst traveling. The rhythm and melody of his music enchants us because it is near to the feeling of *satori*. It should be an encouragement to us to realize that a man can rise to such heights in the course of his daily life. The secret is always to give total attention to whatever we are doing at the moment. Then all life becomes a training in concentration. When *satori* is experienced, joy suffuses us and we feel a great harmony with all that lives. So we may say that the natural laws of life lead us to *satori* but we may hasten the process by intelligently cooperating with it. This state of balance is not emphasized enough by present day Indian Yoga, which tends to seek only for individual spiritual experience. The Buddha was the greatest Yogin the world has known precisely because he went beyond this limited goal to freedom.

Yoga has links with religions other than Buddhism and Jainism. The religion of Zoroaster in ancient Persia incorporated many Yogic concepts and practices and later transmitted these to Judaism when the Persians conquered the Jews during the 4th Century B.C. Stemming from Judaism, Christianity and Islam share some features of the Yogic tradition in common, such as fasting, asceticism and contemplation. It is also probable that Christianity was directly influenced by Brahmanism and Buddhism, for the Mediterranean area had an ancient connection with India. Traders and migrants passed in both directions interchanging ideas and disseminating religious practices, including Yoga. The fundamental principles taught by the Prophet Mohammed and expressed in Islam owe much to Yoga and the Yogic influence is even more obvious in some of the "folk" religions of the Middle East. The debt to Yoga is most clearly seen, however, in the Islamic sects known as the *Dervishes*, for the spiritual attainment of these men has had a profound effect upon the rest of Islam. Many religious teachers in all parts of the world have given me confirmation for my belief that all religious discipline stems originally from Yoga. At first I doubted this but after experiencing the spiritual practices of all the major religions, I have come to see that it is true. Whether I was in a Catholic monastery, amongst a group of *Dervishes* in a cave, in a Tibetan monastery, or a temple of Taoism, Shingon, Zen or Jodo Shinshu, I found that Yoga is the common denominator.

Yoga is thus the Mother of all religious discipline but, unlike most religions, it does not have a sacred scripture. It is for this reason that no theological or philosophical controversies disturb Yoga. Yoga has survived for six thousand years because it consists solely of practical disciplines and, whilst Yoga may be found in all religions, it has no exclusive connection with any one religion. So we can say that Yoga, is, in this sense, beyond religion because its principles are universally and eternally true.

5. The God of Yoga

Theoretically, religion is a distillation of wisdom and experience and its function is to teach us the most vital truth about life. The most vital thing for each one of us is life itself, yet religion has very little to say about that. For Yoga, however, the very activity of life is sacred and the most religious activity is to harmonize ourselves with the Life-Force. Yoga is a life science which stimulates us to full activity, gives us a superior way of living, and provides a practical philosophy.

It is commonplace for the proponents of each religion to claim that only the God they worship is the true God. This very claim reduces religion to idolatry and so they lose the most precious thing by wanting to keep it exclusive. About ten years ago, when I was in America, I was invited to lecture in a "whites only" church at Long Beach. I was to address the members of a biblical seminary on the subject of religion. Before beginning, I set my hosts the notoriously difficult task of defining the word "religion" and so they produced three large dictionaries. The first offered no definition at all and they were unable to deny that this raises profound problems for a priest. The second dictionary said that—"Religion is to enter into union with God"—yet when I asked them to explain to me how to do this, they could not. So many people today are content to substitute abstract theological discussion for real spiritual experience, but this is quite opposite to the basic thrust of Yoga. In view of the fact that the word "God" was continuously on their lips, I next asked my friends to show me God. Of course, they were unable to do this and felt some considerable embarrassment when I pointed out that they were claiming to be experts in what they could neither define, practice nor produce! To resolve the problem, I asked two of the priests to join me on the stage and to sit face to face on two chairs. "It is actually quite easy to see God," I said, and banged their heads sharply together. Their instant reaction was to cry "Ouch!," draw in their breath and adopt a very different posture! I think they forgave me when I explained the point of my actions, for their reactions were the activity of God. Neither the exclamation, the in-drawn breath, nor the movement of hand to forehead were premeditated but manifested clearly the wisdom of God. These changes were both instantaneous and totally appropriate and, although we might tend to devalue them as "just natural," they are actually miraculous. Pain is felt only where there is life and makes us aware of what we are not normally aware: the Life Force which is present within us. The Life-Force is God flowing through our minds and bodies and the way of consciously implementing God's will is Yoga. Thus Yoga teaches us exactly how to relate our individual life force to the cosmic Life Force in order to conform to the eternal law of balance and harmony.

To maintain balance in mind and body is to preserve balance with the universe. This is the natural law and it is because it has been largely forgotten in modern times that there is so much unhappiness and loss of humanity. Although our civilization is the product of science and technology, there is a failure to maintain fully rational policies even in medicine and engineering, for example. Human nature always tends towards the irrational and will complacently accept the fact that some part of a general theory is missing, causing too much emphasis to be placed upon one aspect to the detriment of the whole. Thus there has been little attention given to the social cost and morality of many large scale engineering projects which have caused grave environmental pollution. Nor can medical science escape the charge that dangerous new drugs have been, all too commonly, administered irresponsibly.

It is the central fact of our times that most people have lost their natural balance and health due to the artificiality and stress of living in modern society. Yet very few people realize it because, due to human habit-forming tendencies, they uncritically assume that they are living naturally. It is only when we consider our normal life-style from the detached vantage point provided by the Dōjō, that we can see the truth. Although modern society appears brilliant and sophisticated on the surface, it ruthlessly sacrifices its members in many ways: hence the need to practice Yoga. Visitors to the Dōjō are frequently appalled to find that a considerable percentage of the students are regarded as incurable by the orthodox medical profession. The Dōjō provides for these people as well as for those who are conventionally regarded as being in good health. Our daily task is to repair twisted bodies and minds and to restore them to some degree of normality. Serving and teaching is thus a sacred work through which we learn to replace self-interest with love. It is a process of becoming less self-centered and more centered in the total situation which includes the sufferings of others. This way of living brings true joy and I believe that it is the true teaching of Yoga. We have to accept that we are responsible for others and that their pain is our pain. The problems created by modern social conditions have to be faced and solved by our own unaided efforts.

Yoga is not merely a technique to gain limited objectives, nor is it characterized by end-gaining. Yoga makes man divine in the sense that it releases his power to heal himself, but if it heals difficult physical conditions, or gives longevity, these are really secondary. Most people fail to understand that disease, as such, doesn't really exist. If we practice the wisdom of living entirely in the present, we gain a positive and active mind and disease will depart. Disease is really a sign of the body's active bid to recover its natural condition, which we call health. Properly regarded, therefore, disease is actually the most valuable opportunity to gain self-knowledge and to make progress towards self-realization and sanctity. During the relatively few years of its existence, the Okidō Dōjō has helped more than ten thousand chronically ill or mentally disturbed people to heal themselves. Yoga activates the natural power of self-healing so that it is not really Yoga which heals them so much as their dedication and committment to practice. Through serving others and seeing their suffering, even the seriously ill person develops a sense of gratitude and thankfulness for his own relatively good fortune. The life of exercise, good diet and cleanliness is illuminated by a positive mind so that people move, almost inevitably, towards health and self-knowledge. It is by learning independence and self-reliance that we can arouse the power of self-healing as well as *bussho*, or natural wisdom. Through these, we can approach *satori*.

It was my personal experience of fighting cancer for thirteen years which taught me these valuable truths. It made me realize, most clearly, the fact that I am alive and that this is a great privilege which the Sacred is continually bestowing upon me. Cancer compelled me to study Yoga with total concentration, honestly and seriously. I realized that my life is not my own, but a cooperation between the divine spirit in me and the Sacred power behind the universe. To become aware of this cooperation at the highest level is the aim of Yoga. The *Upanisads* sum it up pithily as "That thou art." It is vital that we should practice Yoga totally if we are to make spiritual progress. Yoga will not help if it is merely a minor part of our life: it must become the whole of our life. *Meiso Yoga* sees the whole person and contains everything that is necessary to form a total way of life. Although modern civilization has many obvious merits, it is fatally flawed by the division in thought represented by the arts and the sciences. The result is an absence of wholeness and an emphasis on partial truths which amounts to an unnatural imbalance of mind. The frustrations and diseases of civilized society are the inevitable consequence. Yoga, if it is properly understood, can heal this condition through its philosophy of totality and its advocation of acceptance, non-attachment, unification, and freedom.

Chapter 2   Basic Training

1. The Eight Stages of Yoga

Many people think that Yoga means the *asanas*—those physical contortions which look impossible for anyone with bones in their body. Of course *asanas* are an important part of Yoga, but are by no means the whole. In Okidō, there is no special emphasis placed on any one kind of exercise, since I believe that all are important. It is actually very difficult to be a complete "all-rounder" and to do every part completely, yet we have little choice. If Yoga is allowed to degenerate into the *asanas* alone, then circus acrobats would be the best Yogins.

Unfortunately, it is these extreme poses of Yoga which have caused most misunderstanding. It is true that we can greatly increase our flexibility through practicing the *asanas*, for it is amazing what self-training can accomplish. Yet that is not Yoga. I want to emphasize that the true aim of Yoga is to evoke the innate ability to make balance, which implies that we become open to that universal energy called *Prana*, or *Ki*. Yoga changes the quality of consciousness and brings true joy as distinct from momentary happiness. This is a deeply religious experience, yet it is only by actually engaging in the practice of Yoga, as distinct from merely reading about it, that this level can be reached. Yoga purifies, adjusts and raises the level of consciousness and *all* practices which can help to bring this about should be utilized.

The test of true Yoga is to look at the mind and body of the teacher. "Through their fruits you shall know them." In Yoga, the basic training includes meditation but meditation is also the ultimate goal. Indeed, there are many practices which are part of the basic training but they cannot be graded according to difficulty. Proficiency in Yoga cannot be graded because it is a spiritual training. It is impossible to award ranks, or *dan*-grades, as in the

Martial Arts. In Yoga, all practices are necessary for it is the combined training which is most effective and we cannot afford to reject anything. Although *Patanjali* analyzes Yoga into eight stages this is only for purposes of explanation: all of them should be practiced together and not one after the other. Those people who use Yoga just for exercise, or relaxation, or to calm the mind, fail to understand the aims of Yoga. These are:

(a) To bring us to greater humanity.
(b) To awaken in us the mind of service.
(c) To bring us to true meditation.

I can say, quite definitely, that most of the Yoga that is taught today is not real Yoga. That is because it neither pursues nor maintains these aims. Furthermore, because most Yoga is unbalanced, it actually harms people by developing them one-sidedly. If a human being can live strictly according to nature he will have health and happiness, because such a way of life is balanced. One-sided training makes people unbalanced and neurotic. The blessing of good health comes to those who find their own individual life-style and adhere to it. It does not come to those who merely accept this or that ready-made system.

Many people will enthusiastically recommend such "cure-alls" as water, this or that herbal medicine, raw vegetables, brown rice, an exclusively alkaline diet, or fasting. Each of these prescriptions for health contains some truth but each is one-sided. Inevitably, they result in imbalance and create abnormality. The proponents of these "cures" claim miraculous successes, yet the same treatment could worsen the condition of, or even kill, another person. However, that possibility is usually ignored. Yoga opposes one-sidedness, attachment and over-dependence upon any one thing, whether it is a remedy or a form of exercise. My advice is always to seek the truth by yourself, not to rely exclusively upon anything, yet not to fall into skepticism. The body-mind system possesses the innate power of recovering health and the Yogic method of curing human ills aims at stimulating it.

Many of today's exercise systems are also one-sided, or biased, for we need to include many different kinds of movement and activity. In exercise, as in much else, the best method is to combine the wisdom and experience of both East and West. Many Western exercise systems must have been created by people who were themselves unbalanced and, unfortunately, they attract and perpetuate unbalance in students. The wisest policy is, therefore, to play many different kinds of sports and not to over-specialize in any single activity.

Recently, in Japan, certain medical drugs have been prescribed and have afterwards been recognized as killers. This is an extreme example, yet a medicine which can apparently improve one condition can, at the same time, cause harm elsewhere in the body. Some chemically synthesized medicines create depression, for example, and forms of ill-health. Increasingly, those who have not regained health through orthodox treatments are searching for an alternative. Such people often turn to Oriental therapies, but if they are wrongly used or wrongly administered, even such traditional ways will only make the patient worse. Occasionally, however, a miracle can happen, such as those cases of healing which have resulted from eating brown rice. Yet we must recognize that even brown rice, if unwisely eaten, can be harmful to the body and the nervous system.

I have tried most of the health systems and cures in the world and I have seen the good and bad in each. My cumulative experience crystalized as Okidō, which is the Yoga of "seeking the way." It embraces aspects of Indian Yoga, Zen, chanting, worship, and the Chinese philosophy of Yin and Yang. Because of its breadth, it harmonizes perfectly with modern philosophy and medical science and, unlike many narrowly based exercise systems, it does not force people beyond their capabilities. Okidō thereby excludes negative and harmful aspects by being broad and flexible.

When I lived in a Yoga Ashram in India, the Guru said, "Don't do anything unreasonable and don't waste your energies." To be natural in all we do is vital and Yoga seeks to raise vitality to the highest level in order to give full, joyful expression to the Life Force. It also shows us the way to harmonize the individual and universal expressions of the Life-Force in *satori*. The first aim of Yoga is, however, to regain and strengthen natural balance and harmony.

It is sad that many people destroy themselves through severe, obsessive training. When the uninitiated see Yoga, it too can appear unreasonable. This is especially true of the practice of fasting, but Yoga is never unreasonable and always gradual in spite of appearances. An initial fast begins with two or three days on a reduced diet followed by three to five days without food. The maximum overall length of the fast should not exceed ten days. In my own case, by gradually increasing the length of the fast, I was able to reach sixty-five days without any harmful effects. What looks severe to others is actually quite reasonable when approached in this gradual way. If people have a positive attitude and Yoga training is done correctly, it will be both beneficial and peaceful. When the mind is calm and all is seen clearly, the training is mentally enjoyable and spiritually rewarding. There is a wonderful sense of detachment, lightness and peace. Those who practice fasting with this frame of mind actually enjoy what they are doing and so it is far from unreasonable. But if we fast fearfully, or reluctantly, it can do more harm than good.

The essential thing is to continue the training without being extreme in any way. The purpose of Yoga is not to establish world records, to indulge in sensationalism, or to demonstrate any kind of political protest. A person who is fasting is not interested in seeking sympathy, or causing others to worry, for he is practicing Yoga. Therefore, we ought to encourage such people, for by purifying themselves they cumulatively purify the entire world.

According to *Patanjali*, the eight stages of Yoga are as follows:

1. *Yama* — The universal moral laws.
2. *Niyama* — The ethical code for the individual.
3. *Asana* — Right posture and movement.
4. *Pranayama* — Correct breathing and diet.
5. *Pratyahara* — Control of the senses.
6. *Dharana* — Concentration practice.
7. *Dhyana* — Zen training for *Mu*-mind.
8. *Samadhi* — Oneness or unification.

The last three stages are known collectively as *samyama* and lead to the attainment of full Enlightenment—the religious ecstasy and joy which arises from the highest and most pure state of consciousness. I will explain the eight stages in more detail, especially the fourth and the last three. Enlightenment is the essence of *Meiso Yoga*.

2. The First Stage

Yama—the way to establish the correct mental attitude.

The *Yoga Sutra* defines Yoga as—"Stilling the fluctuations of the mind." This means controlling the mind until it becomes calm so that *satori* can arise. In order to break long established patterns of associative thought, concentration and self-control have to be practiced. The first and second stages of the Yogic path teach the attitude of mind necessary for practice. *Yama* is basic morality which guards the mind from disturbance by moods, emotions and desires. It is the practical application of principles to Yoga which are common to all religions. Whilst it is true that morality is thereby rendered merely prudential, in that we perform moral actions only because it is prudent to do so, it is a higher prudence which is at work and not self-interest.

All religions contain prescriptions for the moral life. Buddhism has its Five Precepts; Moses mediated the Ten Commandments to Judaism and these were later inherited by Christianity. The Christ's Sermon on the Mount and the Ten Stages of Kūkai's Shingon Buddhism are both expansions, or developments of earlier formulations. A similar process took place in Yoga and the end result was *Patanjali*'s Eight Stages in the *Yoga Sutra*. Of these, the first two, *Yama* and *Niyama*, are particularly concerned with morals. The *Yoga Sutra* gives five precepts under *Yama:* non-violence, truth, non-stealing, continence and non-coveting. These are the moral laws which have been found necessary in all human societies. There is therefore a close correspondence between them and the Five Precepts of Buddhism: non-violence, non-stealing, non-lying, continence, and abstaining from intoxicating drink or drugs. These Buddhist Precepts are very ancient and were originally intended for monks living together in groups. Later, they were expanded into a code of more than two hundred rules to regulate daily life in the monasteries. Shingon's Ten Stages add to these basics as follows: non-violence, non-stealing, non-lying, continence, no intoxicants, non-slandering, non-exaggeration, non-coveting, non-anger, and non-resentment.

In *Yama* and *Niyama*, the emphasis is on a life which will conduce to purity of mind, calmness and stability—in other words on factors of mind training rather than on a morality governed by divine authority. If you disregard *Yama* and *Niyama*, you will pay the price of uneasiness of mind in addition to any penalties which may be imposed by society. The first point about Yoga's Precepts is that they are a natural morality which prohibits only those things which are opposed to spiritual development. The second point is that, whilst religious Commandments are given imperatively and backed by the full weight of authority, Yoga's Precepts form an autonomous morality which is self-imposed. This reveals the basic optimism of Yoga.

In Greek philosophy there are a variety of moral codes based upon different principles. Epicurus taught that man should depend fully on his rationality and follow a moral life in order to preserve a balanced mind. This way of justifying morality by basing it on practical considerations is similar to that of Yoga. The difference is that this was the conclusion of Epicurus' reasoning, whereas in Yoga morality is the starting point of practice. Because of this, Yoga does not end in a negative and selfish life-style, but motivates men to repay their debt to society with interest. Yoga involves leaving society at some stage and so looks selfish and life-denying. Through training, however, you learn to serve society far more efficiently and to bring to it the incalculable benefits of balance and peace.

The aim of *Yama* and *Niyama* is the stabilization of spirit and is the first essential step on the way to *satori*. It begins the process of creating that unshakable stability which is completed when we experience that deep sense of oneness with the universe. *Yama* also has a deep and eternal meaning which is difficult to explain even by the use of similes. The best understanding is given by the Christ's profound Sermon on the Mount. It tells us that the old law of moral retribution is ended and that "an eye for an eye" can no longer be the basis of a satisfactory morality. Instead we should love our enemies, turn the other cheek when abused and not hesitate in giving all we have to help others. It amounts to precisely the same autonomous morality and spirit of all-inclusive love and self-giving which illuminates the Precepts of Yoga.

Because Yoga has no Founder and scarcely any written teaching, it has never developed a dogmatic orthodoxy and has never been in conflict with other religions. Yet there have been many great men in Yoga, such as the Buddha, Patanjali and Mahatma Gandhi. You can read what each of them had to say about morality, but you will reach a complete understanding of *Yama* only if you reflect upon the Precepts in the course of actual Yoga practice. *Yama* are not like the Ten Commandments, for they are not obligatory and, in fact, you can originate your own morality if you wish. The point is to preserve a clear and active mind and you may be able to achieve this by observing only one or none of the Precepts. The people who can successfully do this are rare, however, so that Yoga continues to teach the basic Precepts to assist the majority of people to attain self-respect, integrity and strength.

3. Niyama, The Second Stage

Niyama is concerned with purity of mind, for purity rewards us with calmness and optimism. There are five main aspects of *Niyama* and they are all important for the beginner to incorporate into his way of life. They are: cleanliness, satisfaction, ardor, study, and worship.

Cleanliness is not merely external hygiene, although this, too, is important. Cleanliness also means to expel any impure thoughts which are already in the mind and to guard against the entry of any new ones. The mind which aspires to attain *Meiso Yoga* must not be allowed to be disturbed by desire. It is, of course, easy to ridicule purity of mind, yet most people experience it and appreciate it at times. For example, what is nicer than the clean feeling of getting up early on a summer's morning and going out into the sunshine and refreshing breezes? The mind is very pure at such a time, once tiredness has been dispelled. We can sometimes retain this pure mind all day if we refrain from artificial stimulation of the mind and body.

I am very fond of an old Japanese poem which goes:

"My breath was taken away by the beauty of the simple white Porcelain vase in which I fetch cold water from the river in the early morning."

Inevitably, this poem loses a lot in translation, but I hope that the reader can appreciate something of the thoughts and feelings it conveys. The purity and coolness of white porcelain and fresh spring water; the beauty of line of a simple vase against a background of green willows immersed in the early morning mist—all these images are called to mind. If we can capture the purity and integrity of such thoughts and throw off skepticism and desire, we can attain *satori* and become the master of our life. Pure mind can see the wonder of life; we should try to encourage and preserve it.

Satisfaction is the emotional tone which accompanies satiation, or the attainment of a goal. When we have had enough we feel physical satisfaction, but this feeling is only temporary and it vanishes as soon as desire again raises its head. The only true satisfaction is that which fills a mind which has few desires—the satisfaction of renunciation. Satisfaction is thus a teaching which points towards contentment. If the mind is wholly occupied with getting and gaining, there is no peace, for the acquisitive mind is self-perpetuating and endless. When true satisfaction and contentment arise, the mind becomes calm. As Mencius said—"To cultivate the mind, there is nothing better than to lessen desire." The condition of desirelessness is like a sea of clouds in the autumn sky. The air is fresh, clean, bright, still and cool. The clouds are high, white and fluffy. There is great purity in such conditions.

Confucius defines ardor as that mental disposition which arises in the mind when everything is clearly settled. When we know where we want to go and what we want to do we can pursue our objectives one-pointedly and with spirit. When there is true ardor the body will be right according to heaven, or nature, and you will be in good health. When ardor is established in the mind there is the state which the Buddhist texts call *anjinryume*—we know the will of heaven, preserve a calm mind in all circumstances and are not disturbed by trivial details. Ardor means that you are not impelled to action by emotion; that you can act purposefully but not be driven to react by your feelings. If we always act from a mind which is centered and full of ardor, then we clearly know the difference between right and wrong and will always choose the right.

Study and learning means to see everything as it really is, to think correctly and to distinguish the truth. It also means to study and to realize the self. Unless we make a sincere effort to reject illusion in all its forms and to correct misunderstandings, we will easily be swept away by the flood of the emotions. Pleasure, anger, sadness and laziness will overwhelm us sooner or later. Without self-control and self-discipline, human beings can soon become like animals and slide down the slippery slope to moral degradation. The study of the self implies analyzing our own motives and reactions and learning to be free from our projections. By projecting our feelings and desires onto the environment we create the same situations again and again. Only when we learn to let things be can we become truly creative.

Worship is natural when we realize that God is within. The God of Yoga is Life, the Life-Force which inspires and animates all beings and which is the driving force of the universe. It is important for everyone to think deeply about this. Yoga seeks to unify the content and direction of mind continuously. To worship God in Yoga is to deepen your thought about life and to maintain the purity of the mind's contents and its direction. As I have often said, Yoga is the religion of practice. Only in *Niyama* do we rely on words to some extent, for by teaching the precepts which govern our behavior, we make the basis for pure mind.

In the succeeding sections of this book I shall explain the rest of the eight stages of Yoga. The third and fourth stages relate to training the body by means of postures and breathing. The fifth stage is concerned with attaining autonomy of consciousness, whilst the sixth and seventh stages are the mental disciplines leading to Enlightenment. *Satori*, the eighth stage, is the union of the divine in man with the universal divine, the awesome power of the Sacred. In writing about Yoga, it is always difficult to give adequate expression to this essentially practical religion in words. Those who do not practice cannot claim to have entered the gate of Yoga. Especially in the early stages of the path, a competent teacher is necessary to set your feet upon the way. Although I am trying to explain all the stages of Yoga in this book, I actually feel that words can bring you only as far as the second stage. Even though I do my best and even though you read about the later stages with great attention and sincerity, you cannot really understand them without concurrent practice.

Most religions end with the formulation of a moral code, but Yoga begins at that point. We should not suppose, however, that *Yama* and *Niyama* are simple because of this. The truth is that our spiritual progress is affected by all the stages of the path from the first one until the last. Our responses to life vary according to our state of mind; our actions are conditioned by our mental state. In Yoga, therefore, the first steps serve to clean, purify, adjust and dispose the mind correctly. This process is powerfully aided by the practices of the third and fourth stages, however, so that even the moral precepts cannot be practiced in isolation or regarded as a self-contained preparation for the rest of the path. In Yoga it is the total life-style and the total mind-body system which are involved from the first.

4. The Third Stage: Asanas and Dōzen

(1) Why human bodies become disordered

Asanas are the way to good physical and mental balance and not merely a form of physical training, as many people seem to think.

The Third Stage: Asanas and Dōzen / 49

Yogasanas increase the stability of body and mind and form part of the *Zengyo*, or Zen training, of Okidō. This training, which teaches correct posture and movement, is also known as *Dōzen*, or mobile meditation. *Asanas* are the beginning of body training, but also include the subsequent stage of *Pranayama*, or breathing exercises. When we do *asanas*, physiological abnormalities can often be corrected and the mind controlled. By exercising the internal organs we can gain good health and cure, or alleviate, even chronic conditions. But the correct practice of *asana* must be related to right diet and good breathing or the results will be either insignificant or actually harmful. For proper exercise, we must follow the rules and do only what is necessary according to our present condition. For example, if someone has a pronounced forward stoop, there can be many possible causes. The condition can only be corrected if we work on the actual cause. Because of this, every person who comes to the Dōjō is helped to find out what is causing his particular problem and then shown the right way resolve it by his own efforts. In the end it is only self-analysis and personal effort which produce positive results. This is what I call the practical way of seeking health. Only this way can be really effective and produce permanent results. Initially, therefore, we need an experienced teacher who understands how the human body is constructed.

Yoga is not just a remedial system, however, but a way of regaining the natural human condition. Human beings have developed their present form over millions of years beginning as animals that walked upon all fours. Our present posture, although mechanically unstable, is a basic stimulation to our development. Without exercise, we cannot keep anywhere near to a healthy, natural condition and so illness develops. In fact, illness is just an indicator that exercise is needed and so the problems inherent in the human condition are a spur to evolutionary development.

If you take up a four-legged posture you will immediately notice certain limitations. Human beings cannot keep the head raised, and cannot look to the side very easily. The muscles of the neck and the skeletal structure are not suited to these tasks and the proportion of our head weight to body weight is much greater than that of any animal. In the case of human beings, our greatest advantage is the size of the brain and our ability to employ it for complex thought. As human posture has become upright, the brain has become heavier and heavier. Yet standing erect also presents us with the problem of keeping the spine straight. Human evolution is just as revolutionary as the development in birds of limbs into wings. Because we learned how to stand erect, our hands were relieved of the work of supporting the body and so were able to develop new functions. There is a close relationship between the dexterity of the hands and the complexity of the brain.

The change in posture to an erect stance has had far reaching results. The spine, for example, is now required to bear very different stresses compared to those originally present. An erect spine must act as a pillar on which are hung the muscles and the internal organs. One of the chief causes of human illness in body and mind is that the internal organs tend to drop because of the gravitational pull of the earth. Mechanically, the human body suffers from a number of "design" weaknesses and we must recognize that, compared to animals, we are unnatural in certain respects. That is why it is necessary to study ourselves and make the best use of our actual present condition. It is a widely accepted theory that erect posture imposes strain on the digestive system and on breathing and blood circulation. This causes poor elimination, lung diseases and blood stagnation.

It took many millions of years for human beings to develop the erect posture. Associated with it are those many differences between human beings and animals which constitute our humanity. It is a fact that a gorilla-like posture actually encourages animal behavior. This is very apparent to me in my work of correcting abnormal posture, for success is frequently accompanied by corresponding personality changes. Even the slightest abnormality of posture can cause emotional and mental instability.

Zen training is aimed at establishing the most stable condition and *satori* means that a human being has attained perfect balance. Those who suppose that Zen is to be found in Zen temples, or that Yoga is to be found in Indian Ashrams, understand neither Yoga

The Third Stage: Asanas and Dōzen / 51

nor Zen. In Okidō, Zen and Yoga are brought together, yet Okidō does not relate to any specific religious sect. The essential spirit of Yoga arises from the fact that it has no Founder and is not exclusively related to any one geographical location or historical situation. In consequence, there are no limits to the Yogic viewpoint, no conflict with other groups and no attempts to obscure the truth. The real Yogic attitude is to discuss all views openly and to guard against attachment to this or that concept. Only a purified mind can do this. The religious ideas of the past are of little use to us today because they are presented as absolute truth and so merely encourage division between people. In Yoga, only facts are accepted as truth for, as I use the word, Yoga means the most stable condition of body and mind. Yoga is not just another of the world's ideologies; Yoga accepts many great men as its exemplars: the Buddha, the Christ and many more.

I have been fortunate to have had much experience of religion. Even as a child I was taught how to sit correctly and how to chant the holy mantras. Later I studied both Western and Oriental medicine, the Martial Arts and many different sports. *Meiso Yoga* is the essence of all my experience; it is an holistic way which demands that we shall train ourselves in every department of life and not only in the Dōjō. Although I am reluctant to differentiate myself from others, a name of some sort is necessary for my system. Okidō is neither Indian Yoga nor Zen and I am not a specialist in the *asanas*. Rather I teach others how to think and how to find the most suitable way for themselves. Through the study of Okidō, you will come to understand all teachings. Okidō is a demonstration of the wisdom of gathering the very best from all religions, philosophies and sciences. The resulting combination is used to bring out the true personality of each individual.

When I was thirty-five, I visited a country where people live to be very old. You may have read newspaper articles about such people and noticed how much interest is taken in the so-called secrets of longevity. The simple truth is, however, that even if we live to be a hundred, our life will have been worthless unless we have made it of value to others. Value cannot reside in oneself alone. When I met the old people of the mountains, I could not help thinking that we really ought to measure life, not in years, but according to service and wisdom. Most people would be very young indeed! More important than death is to die to self-interest, for to lose all is actually to gain everything.

Primitive people do not have much knowledge of the sort we teach in schools. They don't need it for their life is close to nature. When I was living amongst such people in India and along the Amazon, I lived as they did and shared in their deep sense of natural balance. They were very active people although they lived on very little food. They always rested after meals and often laughed and danced happily. That is the instinctive way of resolving stress and preserving a good balance of energy, for it releases fear, fatigue and tension naturally. This experience made me realize just how much natural wisdom civilized people have lost. Modern medicine has lengthened life but our life-style promotes fatigue and ill-health. We seldom engage in communal festivals as our ancestors used to do and so we find increasing difficulty in releasing tension from body and mind. Modern entertainment is no real substitute; television, for example, actually induces stress.

(2) The Character of Yogasanas

The system of *Yogasanas* has been devel0ped by countless people, over many millenia and in various countries. It includes breathing exercises, diet and concentration as well as actual physical postures. Although it has had no permanent connection with any one religion, I am quite sure that Yoga has always been deeply religious. The figure of a Yogin, found at *Mohenjo Dharo*, shows a male figure in a Yogic sitting posture. At that early time, there was no established system of Yoga, for Yoga was just the spontaneous expression of natural wisdom. Not surprisingly, the *asanas* seem to have been modeled on the postures of wild animals. Animals can survive only as long as they can keep in first class condition, for wild life maintains perfect balance and admits no extremes.

Ancient people had many mental images of wild animals because they saw them regularly. I also saw many wild animals when I was in India, South Asia and Africa. I was tremendously impressed by their vitality and flexibility and by the way they move. The life which animates them is so wonderful, beautiful and strong that it makes a sensitive person feel like crying. This quality, seen in tigers and deer for example, is rarely captured in photographs. Amongst the *Yogasanas* are many poses which are actually named after animals, such as the fish, cobra, peacock and cat *asanas*, as well as the breathing exercises named tortoise and crane.

One important feature of *asanas* is that they make us adopt poses which are very different to the ones we do in the course of our daily activities. The inverted postures, such as head stand, are a good example of this and there are many others. As civilization develops, increasingly we make only partial use of the body and, in time, our habitual postures become fixed. Under the general conditions of modern life it is very difficult to regain balance and stability. The continuous stimulation to which we are subjected builds up a high residual tension of which we may not be fully aware. This is cumulative in effect and can lead to chronic fatigue and chronic illness. A limited range of habitual postures is contrary to the natural law of change and balance. *Yogasanas* help us to break our fixed habits of posture and increase our ability to recover balance. The corrective exercises of Okidō are also based upon this principle: that we can eliminate our bad habits consciously and so release ourselves from chronic illness. A natural body is equally developed in every respect and always functions as an harmonious whole.

The unifying center of the body is called *uddiyana* in Indian Yoga, *t'an t'ien*, or *tanden* in China, and *Hara* in Japan. The purpose of all the body training systems was originally to strengthen the *Hara* and the basic principle of movement is to move by *Hara*. The *asanas* teach us to move by *Hara* and also strengthen *Hara*. With regard to the relationship of *Hara* and faith, I will give a detailed explanation later. In *Yogasanas*, all movements should be done by *Hara*, or the abdominal power. In Yoga, *Hara* is sometimes called the seat of God. When we concentrate the whole body power in *Hara* we can begin to regain the natural body. *Hara* power is proportionate to stability of mind and it makes a very real difference to all our movement. Although it does not correspond to any discrete organ or muscle, it can be physiologically located with great precision. The stronger the *Hara* and the more effective the self-healing power of the body will become. There are three aspects to *Hara* power: dynamic, static and mental. A developed *Hara* involves the harmonious cooperation of all three.

(a) The dynamic power of *Hara* means whole body movement. As the ability to tighten the anus increases, power is more easily focused in the big toes, lower abdomen and waist.
(b) The static power of *Hara* is created by correct standing and sitting postures. The neck should be gently extended and the shoulders relaxed. The chest should be spread and the muscles of the back and abdomen stretched upwards and downwards. In sitting, the waist should be pushed forwards so that strength comes to the inner side of the knees.
(c) *Hara* power is related to mental and emotional stability and there is a mutual interaction between these two factors. Concentration and meditation influence from one direction, *Hara* strengthening exercises from another. The two come together in movement meditation, or *dozen*.

Thus the aim of the *Yogasanas* is to increase and unify the power of body and mind, to develop stability and self-control, the ability to adapt, endurance and stamina. By making fundamental changes in the body we can make ourselves better and more effective human beings.

In all the movements of life, and not only in the *asanas*, attention and concentration are essential. Doing and knowing, practice and knowledge, must be brought together. If we grasp the philosophy of the *asanas* and know something of their effects as understood by science, we can easily combine a keen awareness of what we are doing and why we are doing it with movement and breathing. When this way becomes habitual and is followed throughout our daily activities, we will clearly experience the truth that mind and body

The Third Stage: Asanas and Dōzen / 55

are one. If you move tentatively, with awareness and by the relaxing breath of *Hara*, you will have a balance of tension and relaxation. When the *Hara* breathing has become habitual, the ability to maintain the balance of body and mind will arise naturally, and stability will be increased. The basic rules of right movement may be stated as follows:

(a) Make deliberate, controlled movements, not short, jerky ones.
(b) Breathe smoothly, and deeply, not in a series of short gasps.
(c) Keep silence and don't make little grunts and wheezes.
(d) Retain power in the lower part of the body at all times.

The essential point is that, if you move with a strong *Hara*, you will have ample power in the abdomen and spine. This condition has been called "breathing through the legs."

Hara Breathing: You can easily see that even domestic animals breath abdominally and so do primitive people. As we became civilized, there was an increase in self-consciousness and natural breathing changed to thoracic breathing in the chest. People who can walk erect and use their hands also develop their brains. But they form the habit of considering too much rather than responding spontaneously to situations. As the brain of man became heavier, the blood was more liable to gather in the thoracic area and spinal disorders tended to follow. Consequently we changed to chest breathing and the general stability of the body, centered in *Hara*, became weak or non-existent. People in that condition are easily excited and prone to tension in body and mind. This abnormality is clearly reflected in the civilization we have created. The distortions inherent in modern society can be explained entirely on the basis of loss of *Hara* power. Most modern people are over-stimulated and over-excited; they do not radiate calmness and peace. Nor do they possess much ability to concentrate or persevere and tend to give up rather easily. With the loss of *Hara* power, the action of the parasympathetic nervous system is obstructed and the sympathetic nervous system becomes overactive. In other words, the suppressive nerves fail to balance the nerves of action and so there is over-stimulation and over-excitement. If we strengthen the *Hara* and make abdominal breathing habitual, the resulting pressure in the abdomen will stimulate the suppressive nerves. A calming hormone is produced which balances the stimulating hormone produced by the sympathetic nervous system. In this way we can recover not only natural breathing, but also the lost physiological and hormonal balance of the body. The importance of *Hara* is not only for the individual body and personality, but also for the future of the human race.

It is essential to do *Yogasanas* together with breath and concentration because this strengthens *Hara* power and helps you to regain natural health. An *asana* done without breath and mind is not Yoga and, worse, can produce abnormality. *Yogasanas* are *dōzen* because they form a kind of mobile meditation when done correctly. After *asanas* it is very necessary to relax and one of the best ways is to take up the "dead man" pose. Alternate tension and relaxation is the balance of life, the flow of Yin and Yang. When the correct rhythm is present there is also the natural life which is the way to health and to stability of body and mind. Too much hard training, however good, builds up tension and affects you adversely by causing you to lose interest. An imbalance is created and tightness of the body and mind will be the result. *Yogasanas* incorporate a correct balance of tension and relaxation. They help to increase concentration, to develop breathing ability and to center power in the *Hara*.

(3) Asanas as Dōzen

About sanmitsu exercise. In Yoga, the life of body, mind and the whole environment are regarded as one. Physical training is therefore also mental training and, at the same time, a way of heightening the quality of life. *Yogasanas* increase our ability to maintain balance, improve stability of mind and body, and strengthen self-control. They also train us in self-reliance and the knack of finding the most efficient way of using the body in all our daily activities. The basic principle of Yoga is the unity of body, mind and breath, which is known as *sanmitsu* in Zen. Whilst there are many specific uses of the *asanas*, the common purpose of all of them is to create *sanmitsu*. Unity, stability, harmony, concentration, contentment, adaptability, and recovery power are all heightened.

In Yoga, we practice in order to lower the center of gravity of the body. From a developed *Hara* comes good breathing and concentration. The natural result is whole body movement. If the body is being abused by partial or unbalanced usage, it will react by tightness and pain. If the wrong usage is continued, the abnormality will become established, causing stress and producing chronic tiredness of body and mind. Illness is the movement of life to correct this condition and restore balance.

How to know yourself through movement: When there is good posture and movement, the hormone balance is restored and mind and body become stable. In this condition, you are naturally calm, have a feeling of well-being, a deep breath, physical fitness, and a normal appetite. Stability, resistance to poisons, and adaptability to circumstances will improve markedly and you will develop the lively, active mind of the warrior. Once you bring the principle of *sanmitsu* into your life, every activity will become part of your spiritual path. In Zen, it is said that the whole of life is a ceremony. This is called *buppo* in Japanese. When you reach this state, the balance of your body and mind may be said to have appeared in your posture, breath and movement. Be sensitive, therefore, to your own condition. If you feel that a certain course of action is abnormal, if your breath is disordered, or if your mind is confused, understand that life is warning you to stop. Once you realize that God teaches you through your difficulties and sufferings, you have entered the first stage of faith.

Self-correction and self-discovery: The *Yogasanas* heal and reveal the problems of body and mind. Difficulty or physical resistance to a specific posture indicates abnormality. Subsequent ability to perform the posture easily shows that the abnormality has been corrected. Abnormalities of this kind come from lack of exercise, but the ability to resist infection and to recover from illness are also lowered. *Yogasanas* characteristically produce a more powerful effect upon abnormal people than normal. For this reason, Okidō contains special corrective exercises, called *shuseiho*, for the treatment of specific abnormal conditions. Yet the most important principle of training is that each person must search for the *asanas* which are most suitable for himself and set his own targets and limits for training.

As a result of Yoga training, you should be able to discover the optimum posture, movements and breathing for any specific activity very quickly. This is the application of natural wisdom to life and, when it is perfectly mastered, a person is said to have attained *satori*. When you really know how to use the body, the way to supreme health is open. From this explanation, you can easily see that you cannot practice Zen discipline as a preparation for *Meiso Yoga* merely by sitting in meditation. In every action, the whole body should be balanced and unified. When body, mind and breath cooperate together, you can practice the correct Zen discipline and *Kinen*, or faith, will arise spontaneously. Through this you can reach to *satori* and Enlightenment. In real *Meiso Yoga*, you are not only taught how to sit, but also how to perform every posture and movement. This is the important difference between *Meiso Yoga* and other trainings, including Zen. In *Meiso Yoga* the whole body is equally developed and brought into full cooperation with a unified mind. At first, Zen didn't teach people that "just sitting" is enough. The Chinese are active and hard-working people and the character of Zen in China was also active and practical. In Japan, it was mainly the *samurai* who patronized Zen. They trained themselves in eighteen Martial Arts as a matter of routine and were extraordinarily active people. The *samurai* ideal was to develop the whole body at the same time practicing *zazen*. The Zen of today would surely be incapable of serving such people.

5. The Fourth and Fifth Stages: Diet and Breath Control

(1) What human beings take from the Universe

After the stage of *asana* we come to *Pranayama* which means the correction of body and mind and the attainment of self-control through diet and breathing. *Asanas* make such a strong impression on many people that they think that all else is subordinate, but through training in the Dōjō it becomes apparent that physical exercise is really no more important than diet and breathing. The two are actually complimentary but, if I was asked to say which is most important, I'd say diet and breathing because for most people they are the more difficult to master. In *asanas* we learn how to use the body and maintain postures but diet and breathing also develops and improves our vehicle. *Asanas* together with *Pranayama* are a powerful means of changing a body which has become used to an unnatural life-style. Diet is crucial as can be seen from the fact that many Yogins who have returned to normal life lose their balance because of failing to keep to right diet.

In Okidō, we have a religious understanding of diet and breathing in life. Yoga says that all life should be a religious ceremony and this is true especially of eating because, through food, the life of others is added to you. In my explanation of Yoga philosophy, I mentioned the relationship between the individual life and the life of the Universe. Through diet and breath we take in the energy of the greater life and change it into vitality, bones and tissues. Even the chemical processes in the body are not independent but depend upon the action of enzymes which the body obtains from the environment. Diet and breath are two physiological processes which conduct a two-way exchange of materials between the "inside" and the "outside." Yoga speaks of universal life-energy as *Prana*, or *Ki* in Japanese, and through diet we receive the combined *Ki* of heaven and earth. People commonly think of the body and the environment as separate and distinct and this is especially true of Western thought which clearly distinguishes between self and other. But in Oriental philosophy, derived from Yoga, self and other, mind and matter, are regarded as one, harmonious whole. Two famous Taoist teachers, *Lao-Tzu* and *Chang-Tzu*, taught this way of thought and it is also found in the Chinese Buddhist philosophy of *Hwa Yen*, the way of totality. In Japan this became known as *Kegon*. Many folk religions also developed this holistic philosophy in Japan and were known, generically, as *Shingaku*. (*Shingaku* means "mind learning.") One in particular, the *Yomei* school, stressed the need to learn through mind and body. Though we have no surviving literature from the *Shingaku* schools, references to them are sufficient to show the influence of Yoga on the Japanese tradition. As the way of unification, Yoga naturally gives rise to the philosophy of totality.

The Yoga teaching about diet and breath is logical and scientific, yet also religious. The human body is essentially mutable for all its cells are constantly renewed and dead cells are exhaled or excreted and some are consumed by growing cells in the body. Through diet and breath, new materials are supplied to create new cells and maintain the organism. For a considerable part of the life of a human being, bones and tissues are replaced in this way. We should learn to see the body as infinitely changeable and plastic and dispense with the illusion of permanence.

Even such large organs as the stomach are completely renewed within ten years and chronic illness only demonstrates that bad habits and an inflexible mind are preventing the renewal of cells. If this situation is corrected and the natural processes are augmented by Yoga training, any condition can be cured without surgery as long as it has not resulted in a pathological abnormality. This is the basis of my conviction that the body can itself cure all illness if its natural powers are stimulated and trusted. Human bodies are subject to aging and degeneration, but if the natural balance is maintained between ingestion and excretion, inhalation and exhalation, the body will be purified and renewed every few years.

By conscientiously practicing Yoga in our lives we can overcome conditioning and utilize our heredity to the best advantage. To go deeply into the practice of *Pranayama*, however, we must leave behind the theoretical approach to diet and breath. Until you have regularly and consistently practiced *Pranayama* for some time you

The Fourth and Fifth Stages: Diet and Breath Control / 61

cannot appreciate its value. It is quite natural that many people coming to Yoga seek only what is quickly and physically effective, but it is through *Pránayama* that the mysterious union between the individual life and the life of the Universe takes place. Breath and eating are life's supreme ritual because through these functions the individual life is joined to and augmented by myriads of other lives. It requires long practice before we can deeply experience this even though we may readily understand it intellectually. *Pranayama* is one of the bases of *Meiso Yoga* yet if you don't achieve *Meiso Yoga*, you cannot completely master *Pranayama*.

In the eight stages of Yoga, each stage must be practiced both sequentially and concurrently, so to reach the eighth stage we must practice every stage. If you continue to practice *Meiso Yoga* the mind and body become stable and natural and your desires are changed to the minimum. Your taste in food is also changed and the breath becomes deep and harmonious. Now let me explain about food and its relationship to *Pranayama*.

(2) The way of right eating

Right diet cannot be found through studying dietetics or by counting calories. There are three kinds of food, those which are good for the body, the mind and spirit. By experiment we can discover and combine these foods to construct an individual diet which will make the most of our innate abilities. The food which makes you most natural and most spiritual is the most suitable food and each person must find it for himself.

Food is the product of the *Ki* of Heaven and the *Ki* of Earth and when it is eaten, it is changed. Food becomes the blood, flesh, bones and energy of the body so that the body is directly affected by diet as regards both its maintenance and its operation.

Thousands of years of experience have gone into the Yoga teaching about diet which has developed as a result of practical observations of the effect of different foods on body and mind. If we try to live solely on so-called natural foods we find that they, too, can become unnatural. In the times when human society was primitive, men ate quite different foods compared with what we eat today. The basis of their diet was fruits, seeds and roots which they gathered freshly according to need, like animals. With the invention of fire, however, seeds, grasses and plants were cooked and the staple foods of human diet were radically changed. People were able to cook and eat what was inedible before, so that they had more food and began to increase in size. The consumption of meat increased and many ways of storing food were developed. Not only was the range of the diet widened but the number of acceptable locations for human habitation was multiplied. The ability of human beings to adapt to different conditions increased and many new kinds of experience acted as a stimulation, causing the size and complexity of the brain to increase. Human beings became far less dependent upon the environment, for even when natural foods were scarce, or out of season, people could eat stored foods such as rice, wheat and pickles. Thus the range of human diet was enlarged and given greater variety; the quantity of food consumed was also increased as a result of food becoming more abundant. Special foods were developed and preferences for specific foods arose. Some African tribal people of today, who subsist by hunting and gathering, have a life-style which is similar to that of primitive people in ancient times. They are not attracted by our processed foods and don't want to spice their food, or cook it. Most civilized people eat cooked food from infancy and add many unnatural materials in processing and cooking. Because of this, their senses of taste and smell become warped. In animals those same senses are a vital aspect of their self-protection mechanism and, for example, they can determine the suitability of food by smelling, tasting and cooking. Human beings have lost this ability and so Yoga diet is important because it contains those foods which are right for us and increase our natural vitality.

"Suitable" is that which is natural, or unprocessed, or that which makes us more natural. There are two basic kinds of suitable food:

(1) Pulses, nuts such as chestnuts, and various kinds of leaves, herbs and plants.
(2) Wholefoods such as vegetables—whole in the sense that

The Fourth and Fifth Stages: Diet and Breath Control / 63

we should eat the whole thing—roots and leaves.

The ideal body condition is slightly alkaline and people who eat the above kinds of foods can maintain a good balance because they don't alter the natural condition of the blood. Most people today are too acidic because they have a basically wrong view of nutrition. It is drummed into us from childhood that we must have sufficient protein, carbohydrate and fat for a balanced diet as these three factors are said to be essential for health. Most people develop a liking for foods which are heavy in protein and think that meat, for example, is necessary for energy and vitality. In Japan, people eat large amounts of white rice and this, too, makes for an unbalanced diet. In the case of fish, which also forms a major part of the Japanese diet, it is the alkaline parts—the bones and skin—which are thrown away. It is scarcely suprising that the blood becomes too acid—and the consequence is that the nervous system becomes agitated and the organs become abnormal. Such a physical condition makes consciousness dull: the mind is not calm and is liable to anger; we have little energy and develop an gross appetite for food and sex. Most of our difficulties and sufferings are the result of wrong diet and an over-acid condition of the body.

To correct this condition we must neutralize the acid with alkaline foods. The principle agent is calcium which is the mineral contained in the bones of birds, in raw vegetables, seaweed, nuts, mushrooms and fruit. This is the sort of food eaten by the *Sennin*—the Japanese "Yogins" of the mountains. Yoga teaches that one of the *Chakras* is especially important because it converts food into energy—it is *Manipuraka*, the solar plexus. From the point of view of biology, all nutrients must be broken down by enzymes, such as Trypsin Pepsin, and others, in order that the energy may be released from the food and flow from the digestive system into the body. Over eighty enzymes have, so far, been identified and these are contained in the food we eat.

Some foods, such as raw vegetables, nuts, tree buds, milk, yoghurt, pickled vegetables and soy beans are rich in enzymes. Fruit wine is an especially good source. Once, in the high Himalayas, I witnessed a monkey squeezing juice from a fruit into a hollow in a rock. It is quite astounding, but true, that an animal not only knew instinctively that it needed enzymes, but could actually produce an enzyme-rich liquid through fermentation. The character of traditional Japanese food is quite considerably dependent upon the many fermented foods it contains such as *Miso* and I always admire the wisdom of our ancestors in developing such foods.

The structure of the body and its nutritional needs is explained today in scientific terms. This is excellent, so far as it goes, but it leaves many things unexplained. The "diseases of civilization," for example, still defy all our attempts to find either the cause or the cure —as in the case of cancer. It is very dangerous, and foolish, to assume that the type of food most prevalent in modern society is not an important factor in this problem—perhaps the most important one. We consume large quantities of processed and unnatural foods which fail to supply us with the vitamins and minerals we need. The body needs four basic minerals: magnesium, sodium, calcium and potassium. They help to convey the nutrient materials from food into the blood stream and to cleanse toxins out of the blood. Without them the body degenerates rapidly.

For optimium functioning, the human organism requires sodium and calcium in excess of magnesium and potassium. Calcium, especially, aids the transfer of nutrients from the blood stream to the cells of bone and tissues. The kind of food recommended by Yoga contains calcium and sodium primarily and this without benefit of modern scientific knowledge. The correctness of Yogic natural wisdom is always a source of wonder to me.

If you have an excess of magnesium, muscles and bones age prematurely and become weak. If you have excess potassium the toxin expelling function of carbon dioxide in the exhaled breath will be impaired.

Geologically, Japan is low in calcium and so Japanese people need a diet containing other sources of calcium such as small fish, milk, and especially seaweed. European and American people don't need much seaweed and therefore don't eat it, because the earth of those continents is as much as five times richer in calcium than Japan. It is

The Fourth and Fifth Stages: Diet and Breath Control / 65

only natural wisdom which has directed Oriental people to eat seaweed and I see it as a privilege granted by God so that we can maintain the correct balance of minerals in the body.

Yogic food is mainly vegetarian for the body needs to become accustomed to natural food after years of processed food. In any case, only plants can transmute the minerals of the earth into substances which human beings can eat. Once vegetable matter has been digested and broken, the minerals are dispersed and reabsorbed by plants—it is a natural cycle. Animals and plants perform different but complimentary functions in nature and because of this life is maintained. Yogins conclude that it is natural for human beings to be vegetarian, especially as they were so in very ancient times. Consequently, Yogic diet minimizes animal foods but, in India today, Yogins eat dairy foods, milk, eggs, as well the skin, bones and internal organs of animals. Sometimes they even eat insects such as grasshoppers, honey and oysters. Even monkeys know better than to eat meat—except for two species and even they were formerly vegetarian.

In America and Europe, rheumatism and similar illnesses are prevalent. They are related to the condition of the nervous system and caused by the excessive consumption of animal food. Meat disturbs the nervous system because it contains nucleic acid.

Rice is traditionally the staple food in the Orient but Japanese people today eat far too much white rice. Moreover the modern Japanese diet includes an increasing amount of sugar and meat and so the body becomes too acid and the blood becomes abnormal. In this condition *bacilli* form in the digestive system and can cause illness.

Animal protein has the disadvantage that it is liable to decompose within the body. Especially if a person is constipated this occurs and the resulting poisons are absorbed into the blood stream causing illness.

We should take care to ensure that all processed foods and condiments are completely excreted and avoid foods containing antiseptics or preservatives as much as possible. We should also be careful to avoid foods produced with the aid of chemical fertilizers, for such foods are unnatural.

From the above remarks you may conclude that there is nothing left to eat! This is good because such a feeling is basic to the right attitude towards diet. Yoga doesn't impose a rigid list of foods because the right food for each person is entirely individual. We may learn what is good and bad in a general sense but the essential thing is to learn to know what is right for you.

The right food varies according to several factors, for example the environment and body condition. In the balanced view deriving from Yin-Yang philosophy, meat *is* right for people living in a very cold climate whilst grains and vegetables are more appropriate in the temperate zones. Until comparatively recently, this totalistic way of thinking has not been known in Europe and America. Fruit, for example, is a Yin food which makes the body colder so that it is right for people living in the South or for those who are suffering from a fever. We need Yin food in summer to cool the body and Yang food in winter to warm it. That is the wisdom of life and it teaches us that fruits are not helpful in cases of bad blood circulation which produces coldness or when the body retains fluids and is subject to swelling. By contrast, children are very Yang and like cold stimulation: it is quite natural for them not to like hot baths and warming Yang foods such as carrots and leeks.

The condition of the body should also determine diet and alkaline foods are necessary when descending from a mountain, after crying, taking exercise, being in noisy places, getting angry, eating meat, taking cold baths, or when living in cold temperatures. These conditions stimulate the sympathetic nervous system and the blood tends to become over-acid. On the contrary, acid foods are necessary when climbing, after laughing, eating boiled vegetables, being in quite places, taking a rest or a hot bath, when the body is warm and after any circumstance which causes you to put power into the *Hara*. This is because these conditions stimulate the parasympathetic nervous system which tends to make the blood over-alkaline.

Other important factors in determining right diet are age and sex, but the food which helps the body to recover its natural condition of health and which enables us to improve our performance in a given

The Fourth and Fifth Stages: Diet and Breath Control / 67

direction are quite different. The foregoing remarks about right diet concern only the latter kinds of food. Now I want to explain about *Seishoku*, or macrobiotic food, which purifies the mind and *satori* food which prepares the body for high spiritual experiences. The ability to recognize these foods is essential for the practice of real meditation.

Seishoku food: The effect of *Seishoku* food is to purify, strengthen and calm the mind—in sum: to make the mind sacred. To recognize it you must have a mental attitude consisting of *gratitude* to all who have contributed their efforts to creating the food, including the plants themselves; an *awareness* that life is maintained only by the sacrifice of life and a sense of *service* to others. It is one of the principle laws of the universe that there is a total harmony and cooperation between all things. All forms of life are affected by our physical actions and psychological condition, and we by theirs. Each person should take full responsibility for what he does, feels and thinks and, if he develops his sensitivity in this direction, the plants themselves will tell him what to eat.

Satori food: *Satori* means to become one with the object of your attention and to become one is love. If, for example, you develop a deep respect for your work, you will become one with it and you will receive inspiration about what to eat in order to obtain the greatest value from the work and to work creatively.

The Dōjō Life: In spite of the explanation given here, the reader may still fail to understand the principle of right food. The best way is to come and live in the Dōjō. We get up at 5.30 A.M. and, after various kinds of exercise, the first meal is served about noon. The diet consists of natural foods such as brown rice, wild grasses, beans, pickles, raw vegetables and seaweed—and the menu is different every day. To make balance is to follow the natural law and this means that we should not simply eat everything which is served, but be selective. The person who is accustomed to Dōjō life comes to know what is suitable for himself and eats only individually right food.

68 / BASIC TRAINING

Before commencing a meal or any other training we make *gassho* by placing the hands together and repeat a solemn pledge. In the case of the training in right diet we say:

"Nutrition means to take only what is right and to reject unnecessary things. I possess the inner wisdom which tells me what is good for me to eat and what is bad. From this time forth I will try to respond only to the inner wisdom."

About 6.30 P.M. a bowl of *soba*, or noodles, is served as the second meal of the day. We do not necessarily require it but at first we fear that we will injure ourselves by not eating enough. After being in the Dōjō for about a week, however, we come to realize that the food provided is enough even for hard training and will feel fully satisfied. The body and mind will work well and we begin to experience a new power.

Modern dietetics often stipulates 2,400 to 3,000 calories per day as essential for an adequate diet but this is quite untrue. The volume of food consumed is not important—if it was, all the people in the Dōjō would collapse due to lack of calories. Of course the concept of calorie content is important and cannot be ignored but we should not make it into an inflexible rule to which we subordinate our nature. The truth is that the amount of calories which the body can derive from food is dependent upon our physical and mental condition. When it is in good condition, the human organism can extract more calories from a given amount of food, or the same number as previously, when it was not in good condition, from a smaller amount. In health, this ability is heightened whilst in a degenerate state even special high calorie foods normally given to invalids can become virtually poisonous. My own consumption of food is small and I sleep only for three hours at night, yet I teach and take exercise in the Dōjō along with my students. After they have gone to bed I am usually busy writing in my study yet I don't lose weight or catch colds. Before Yoga training became an essential part of my life I suffered from tuberculosis and intestinal cancer. I was thought to be a doomed man, yet now I am active and feel full of vitality all day long. My body is basically no different to any other but the right diet and life-style makes a profound difference. If we eat a balanced diet and if the digestive system can extract the maximum nutrition from everything we eat by virtue of a good general condition, a little food is adequate. Yoga training is freely begun and freely continued. It teaches self-control not only for your own benefit but also for the good of others. Through Yoga you become master of yourself and can improve your health and personality by your own efforts. This is the very reason for existence and we must conform to it always by learning and doing. Therefore only two roles are possible, that of the leader and that of the follower. You will realize the truth of this if you think about your own experience. Good and evil are relative values and so the opinions of others should not be allowed to prevent you from developing your own individuality provided only that you do them no harm. To become fully yourself you must develop your own way of feeling, thinking and doing and this is why people come to the Dōjō.

Few people understand that only you can resolve your own problems because you, yourself, have made them. Consequently I teach people not to rely upon others to save them. Yoga should train us to be ourselves. Even in the Dōjō, you will not solve your problem without practical participation. In the Dōjō, individuality is encouraged in many ways even to the extent of asking people to select their own rewards and punishments. We must learn to be ourselves, develop integrity and a sense of responsibility for others. That is Yoga. Our natural sensitivity has been impaired because of wrong diet and an unnatural life-style since infancy. One aspect of this is that we have lost the ability to know which food is best for us. In the Dōjō we live a specific life-style in order to resuscitate those parts of human nature which have become dormant or atrophied. We cut-off our bad habits, for example, by fasting and continue on a diet of natural food. Fasting is just one of the methods employed for purification but the most important key for unlocking our sensitivity is the way of breath. If you make the breath natural, all else follows. Your sensitivity will become natural and excessive or unnecessary desires will fall away. An important part of breath training is *Zazen*, the practice of sitting and breathing correctly whilst concentrating on the breath. It is very effective and soon enables people to know what is the correct food for them.

Why is it that Yoga, which is both a philosophy and a living religion, believes that the body is so important and trains it so strictly? Without health we can neither practice meditation nor attain *satori*.

Few people really know what the essential features of health are, or what factors are involved. Health is, precisely, that condition in which a human being has full sensitivity and in which all his faculties are operating fully. To actively work towards this condition is to cure illness and to develop maximum health. It is the first stage of the way to *satori*.

Satori is that state in which wisdom and ability, having each been developed to the utmost, now become one. Total concentration on any one activity with the motive of gaining *satori* is a way of Yoga. Anything and everything you do should be done completely and to the best of your ability. Yoga can therefore be understood as a way of training which combines medicine, psychology, philosophy, religion, and the wisdom of life—which are all needed in the development of a human being. But Yoga is a holistic concept for, even though you may practice *Zazen* and prayer all day, you will not gain *satori* if your blood is abnormal.

In the Dōjō *Danshari* is done to promote calmness and generate right feeling and thought. *Danshari* provides the basis on which the free man can stand by releasing him from all attachment, conscious and unconscious. In fact it means to renounce and gain detachment from everything negative in our lives. When a person's entire life is pervaded by *Danshari* then he is living like a *samon*, the Yogins of old. In Japanese there is an associated concept called *Shukkedo* which means "going-forth" in the sense of leaving home and family and renouncing everything in the cause of truth. For many people a period of residence in the Dōjō enables them to practice and reap the benefits of *Danshari* and *Shukkedo*.

Every person has the innate ability to control himself but as long as we have bad habits we are powerless. Everything that happens to us, including illness and unhappiness, is the result of our own

The Fourth and Fifth Stages: Diet and Breath Control / 71

actions, but because many of our actions are prompted from the unconscious levels of mind, we cannot avoid them or their consequences. When we can bring these motivations into consciousness we can begin to renew ourselves—and this is the way of self-discovery. To change unconscious motivations, attitudes and habits into the contents of the conscious mind requires stimulation, so Yoga trains us to change, purify, improve and strengthen ourselves. In Yoga, all experiencing and all action must be done consciously. To live consciously, willingly, independently and to engage positively in releasing yourself from negative ways is *Danshari* and *Shukkedo*.

One desire affects another so that, if you can control the desire for food you can also control the desire for sex, possessions and everything else. But, since most people cannot control their desires and emotions, they are led into performing misdeeds and sometimes become criminals or otherwise abnormal. Yet we have to recognize that amongst all our many desires is a basic desire which cannot be renounced completely. We have certain minimum requirements to support life. If we take the opportunity in the Dōjō to renounce desire completely for a limited period we can more clearly see the outlines of our basic desire and so learn to work constructively with it in future. In Yoga we find people practicing fasting, celibacy, the renunciation of wealth and possessions, as well as leaving home, loved ones and society. The aim is always the same, to control desire and, since desire is mental and emotional, there are many ways of doing it. Fasting is the most natural and fundamental training for the control of desire, being practiced instinctively by animals and primitive men who live close to nature. Hence it is quite wrong to think of fasting as something strange or abnormal and before forming any judgment we should try it at least once.

Nowadays the wealthy and influential people of the world don't practice fasting but, in ancient times, even kings and queens undertook the discipline regularly. Through fasting you can re-shape your personality because you can learn how to become detached from all desire. Animals practice fasting when they hibernate and insects do so too when they undergo metamorphosis from the larvae to the chrysalis stage, for example. All life-energy arises from stimulation and the larvae reacts against the stimulation provided by fasting to bring about a complete change of physical form. Of all stimulations, it is fasting which most surely raises the level of vitality and increases the ability to change. In the case of human beings, whose consciousness is more developed than animals or insects, fasting causes the mind to become very clear and often this is accompanied by a profound spiritual revolution. Through fasting, you will appreciate more and more the value of things and experience deep thankfulness for all you receive including your responsibilities and the necessity which drives you forward. By enduring the hardship of fasting you will be strengthened in every way.

(3)   Through fasting you can become detached from desire and know yourself

An understanding of the Yogic teaching about diet is most quickly gained by fasting and practicing mental detachment at the same time. It is necessary to fast many times before you come to the end of Yoga training. The value of these practices for the attainment of *satori* is recognized by all religions. All the great founders of religion, the Buddha, the Christ, Mohammed and Lao-Tzu, attained their greatest spiritual experiences after practicing fasting, detachment from desire and meditation. Nowadays only isolated Yoga groups value fasting and practice it as part of *Danshari* discipline. It must be difficult for many of my readers to understand this teaching because so much importance is placed upon the written word today. But real understanding comes only from direct experience, hence the value of actually participating in the different forms of practical training. To value first-hand experience is the best attitude for learning and it is the way of both Yoga and *Mikkyo*, or the esoteric religious tradition in Japan. It was after he had practiced fasting and meditation in the wilderness for forty days, that the Christ was inspired to deliver his great "Sermon on the Mount." The Buddha also attained his Enlightenment only after long fasting and meditation and Mohammed retired to a remote mountain cave for the

The Fourth and Fifth Stages: Diet and Breath Control / 73

same purpose before receiving the visitation of the Archangel Gabriel.

Taoism is traditionally said to have been founded by Lao-Tzu. He apparently did not retire from the world but taught that we should derive all our nourishment from the mother, which means nature. According to Taoism we should eat only the wild herbs, and fruits and, whenever possible, we should eat the whole plant. Taoism has many points of similarity to Yoga. For example, Taoist teaching is that the human spirit is generated by the body, which is dependent upon diet. If you wish to cultivate the spirit and live longer, you should avoid cooked foods and starch and eat herbs, grains whole root vegetables and fruit. You should, however, eat little in order to keep the digestive organs purified and clean. If you take only these natural foods and regard them as medicines you will not only become calm and peaceful but will find that your physical ability has improved as well.

This is virtually the same as what the Yogic texts of India say, and it seems that, at a time when the wisdom of Yoga was highly esteemed by Indian society, it was transmitted to China. In China it acquired a Chinese style and absorbed a great deal of Chinese wisdom, then it was conveyed to Japan by Buddhism and Taoism. In Japan it became the *Sendo*, the learning of the ancient sage—Yogins, which was a kind of Taoist-related folk religion. It is said that the *Sennin*, the old hermits of the mountains, lived on air and this shows that their basic practice was fasting and breath control. There is a great deal in common between the experience of the *Tao*, *Nirvana*, the mind of *Mu* in Buddhism and *Akarma* in Yoga. Periods of fasting and a diet of natural food have long been the basic factors in the life-style recommended by all the great religions. Some modern religions include fasting too, but a subtle change has taken place. No modern religion advocates the practice of fasting first and foremost for purifying the mind and body but offers it, instead, as a way of healing. Yet the fact is that, in the experience of all the great religious men of the past, healing is only a by-product of fasting, so that the modern religions have gone astray on this point.

In Japanese, there are three words relating to the discipline of fasting, *Mushoku, Zesshoku,* and *Danjiki.* Most people do not clearly understand the difference between these words and so I offer a definition:

Mushoku: Literally "eating nothing." In Japan many people go to special centers to practice fasting. They lie in bed, or watch television but, although they do not eat, their minds are dominated and disordered by the desire for food. This is not true fasting.

Zesshoku: Literally "stopping eating." This is done for clear physiological or scientific purposes, as in hospital when a patient is being prepared for an operation. Again the motive is motivelessness.

Danjiki: Literally "cutting-off." True fasting in which the motive is to gain detachment from all desire whether in thought, word, or deed. Through *Danjiki,* correctly practiced, you can release yourself from the domination of the contents of the unconscious mind, purify yourself and reform your personality. Here the motive is motivelessness.

Danjiki is really a way of developing natural wisdom, it prepares you for meditation and makes meditation flow easily towards *satori.* It is natural to suppose that fasting is just a technique for healing illness, but in fact the greater proportion of the effects are psychological and spiritual. If you train the body in order to raise the level of consciousness you will increase your humanity and that is the real aim of all the different kinds of training. All the great religions have known and practiced this method of spiritual discipline. *Zenshu,* the Japanese religious sect, has a special diet, which they call "food for improvement," to prepare them for Zen training. Taoism places special emphasis on pure natural food whilst in Islam fasting is ritualized and elevated to the status of worship. In Judaism and Christianity, too, there are special periods of fasting and the Jews, especially, prescribe special foods at all times. In all religions the purpose of fasting and giving special attention to diet is to promote worship, meditation and self-reflection.

Even though your purpose is not spiritual and you just want practical results from fasting, it is much wiser to fast in the Yogic way placing the emphasis on gaining detachment from desire. You will not get the full benefits of fasting if you practice according to the narrow disciplines of *Mushoku* and *Zesshoku*. Especially when you earnestly want to practice the real *Danjiki* form of Yoga fasting, you should approach it very gradually. In all religions the aim of meditation is to obtain release from our limitations and the absolute freedom of *satori* in which we can live a fully creative life. But most religions today advise people to undertake these powerful spiritual disciplines without prior preparation of body and mind. This is really only possible for supermen so that, once again, we see the practicality of Yoga which explains the preparation step by step. At this point I don't want to give a detailed explanation of the mental practice of fasting, but will do so later. It is sufficient here to say that if you practice meditation concurrently with fasting it will be a most valuable training in detachment from desire.

(4) The physiological and psychological effects of fasting

Fasting energizes the vagus, or parasympathetic nervous system. It calms the mind and the autonomic nervous center, or *Hara*. The stability of the deeper levels of consciousness which are the seat of the emotions is also improved. Fasting has a similar effect to *Zazen*. Fasting can heal a variety of physiological problems caused by overeating such as diabetes, hypertension, palsy, chronicity, pyelitis, weak stomach and intestines, heart disease, corpulency, suppuration, cancer, contagious diseases and chronic illnesses. Human beings almost always overeat and so their ability to evacuate completely is lowered. The stomach and the intestines become swollen and waste matter is retained far too long in the body. Toxins are formed and the position of the internal organs is changed due to the swelling. The effects of fasting are beneficial in correcting this condition since deposits of unnecessary fat which have accumulated in the body are used up and waste matter is more completely evacuated. The result is that the blood is purified and a natural condition is created in which it is impossible for virus to live in the body. It is for this reason that the wounds of hibernating animals don't fester. It is also the reason why some Yogins who practice fasting remain unaffected when they are injected with what is normally a fatal dose of drugs. If we fast before a surgical operation we lower the possibility of blood poisoning and festering considerably and, furthermore, the rate of healing is speeded up.

Another physiological effect of fasting is to rest the internal organs and generate vitality in them. The natural cycle of life alternates activity and rest rhythmically, yet normally people give their digestive organs no respite whatsoever. It is one of the unique characteristics of Yoga that it teaches us a technique for relaxation and applies it after every *asana*. This alone is a powerful corrective for unbalanced blood conditions and illnesses caused by wrong diet.

The process of fasting: Fasting should be done willingly. When a person decides to fast in the Dōjō a schedule is drawn up according to his mental and physical constitution and condition. During the time of preparation the intestines are purged by means of herbal medicine and the body is adjusted by means of a reduced diet consisting exclusively of fresh vegetables. During fasting special attention is paid to evacuation and stimulation is given by means of cold baths, vigorous toweling, exercise, breathing exercises and the use of an enema. A special feature is the use of natural juices extracted from vegetables including brown-rice and fruits to balance the condition of the person's body.

We should take care that fasting is not attended by fear and an uneasy mind, for it can do more harm than good especially in the case of people who are mentally disturbed or neurotic. If disorders of the mind and spirit occur whilst fasting it is wisest to discontinue. The special diet used at the end of the fast should be eaten and a normal diet gradually resumed.

It is really quite unreasonable to expect the body to put up with being plunged directly into fasting. The first step is to go onto a reduced diet for a few days and gradually enter a total fast. Similarly when emerging from a fast, great care should be taken, for upon this depends whether or not you gain any lasting benefit from the fast. More attention should be given to this time than to the fast itself and you should remember that whatever food you take to break your fast will afterwards be your favorite. Eating too much after a period of fasting has sometimes been known to kill people—so take care.

After fasting, your ability to know what is the right food is increased and, if you eat according to this natural wisdom you will come close to your individually right diet. One of the preconditions for real meditation is to understand the connection between the universe and the body. Another is to understand the real meaning of food and both can be gained through fasting.

(5) Pranayama—Yogic breathing

There are two reasons for doing breathing exercises in Yoga, firstly for healing body and mind and, secondly, for gaining breath autonomy, or conscious breath control. The breath plays the important role of controlling the emotions and of integrating the body and mind. So it is said in all the Japanese arts, especially the Martial Arts, that breath is the vital key to mastery. The breath is the means of preserving mental and physical balance and also controls vitality. If the breath is corrected and controlled, appetites and desires revert to normal. Breath is also the way to improve your ability to recover, it arouses natural wisdom and is the key to meditation. The breath is the expression of life and reveals the real condition of body and mind. Every habitual, unconscious function, such as thinking, seeing, acting and feeling, has its own special kind of breath. Unless you can change the associated breath, you cannot eliminate your negative or undesirable habits.

To attain good breathing habits is also to gain natural health and vitality. Calmness of mind is essential for spiritual experiences such as *satori*. It is because it corrects the breath that *Shuseiho*, Okidō's unique system of corrective exercises, gives such remarkable results. Even chronic illness can be healed if the habitual breathing pattern can be changed. One might say that Yoga begins and ends in breath and both Yoga and Taoism regard *Ki*, or *prana*, as life itself. Human beings forget the natural way of using thoracic and abdominal breathing together, which is the balanced breathing of animals. Primitive people laugh and dance a great deal and breath correctly or naturally. When I was living amongst the primitive tribes of India, I realized how civilized people fail to laugh and relax. In our Dōjō, we chant the Heart Sutra, or *Hannya Shinkyo*, three times every morning and do laughing exercises twice a day. These are excellent breathing exercises and laughter also benefits the body and mind. After active, boisterous laughter, you can feel that the breath has been deepened so that laughing induces power into the abdomen, makes the body flexible and relaxes the mind. Full correct breathing as practiced in Zen is equivalent to laughter.

Correct breathing massages and stimulates the internal organs and, if the breath is deep and strong, the blood improves and the whole body becomes more active. The first reason for disciplining the breath is to control the organs and muscles served by the autonomic nervous system. The involuntary muscles cannot be controlled even by strong will power but the breath can be controlled to some degree and can be the mediator. The second purpose is to control the mental and emotional condition. The breath changes before emotional and physical changes occur. For example, there is an intake of breath before crying and when the breath becomes long and quiet, we become calm. If you practice conscious breath control and develop good breathing habits you will be able to change the pattern of your breathing at will and so control your emotions and mind.

The necessity of exhalation and breath retention: Crying, singing and laughing induce a long breath and result in calming the mind. A person who is ill, or in agony, should try to laugh and sing as much as possible. When we practice *Kumbhaka*, or retain the breath, all the energy of the body is concentrated in the lower abdominal area, or *Hara*. The ability to keep your balance and general stability will be improved. Hard work and exercise induce *kumbhaka* naturally but, since few people today are as active as their ancestors, we need to practice *kumbhaka* often.

The Fourth and Fifth Stages: Diet and Breath Control / 79

The rhythm of the breath: Will, strength and the speed of action depend upon the rhythm of the breath. If we strengthen the breath we make the will stronger and the movement more brisk. Inhalation produces physical tension while exhalation brings about relaxation. The practice of *pranayama* is the use of special breathing exercises to change the strength and rhythm of the breath to produce the changes and attain the condition you desire. It is aided if you carry a strong mental picture of the goal and make use of appropriate *Yogasanas*, or poses. Through this process ways we can gain self-control and become what we want to be.

In *Shuseiho*, or corrective exercises, most of the *asanas* are accompanied by exhalation so that tension, tiredness and discomfort are decreased. When you enjoy doing something, exhalation and *kumbhaka* occur naturally and so power flows to the *Hara*. If we do things unwillingly and negatively it is damaging to health and, conversely, all our life is healthy exercise if we enjoy it. It is a fact that, if you are healthy, you don't need exercise but, since we cannot be completely certain about it, it is wiser to do exercise than not to do it! Stamina comes when a strong, deep breath continues rhythmically and naturally. If you do something reluctantly the breath becomes weak and shallow and you'll soon be tired. Details of *pranayama* breathing exercises are given in my book *Practical Yoga*.

(6) The Fifth Stage—Pratyahara

Pratyahara is training the mind to look within and suspend the normal function of the senses of receiving information from the environment. It is very difficult to accomplish this only through mental training so we begin with a physical method. Close the eyes and cover them and the ears using both hands. This doesn't eliminate sound completely and you can give complete attention to the reduced sound. After some time you will notice that the internal resonance, or "singing" in the ears changes. The next step is to cover only the eyes and, once you can give uninterrupted attention to sound, you can focus on the inner sounds at will. Generally, concentration is understood to mean the ability to focus the mind on one fixed point, but the concentration practiced in *Zazen* is quite different. It is the spreading of attention so that concentration is moving with life. When this is achieved we see things in their wholeness without losing awareness of any single object. *Pratyahara* leads us towards *satori* in which subject and object, the knower, the knowledge and the known, become one and coalesce totally.

Chapter 3 Meditation

1. The Width and Depth of Yogic Meditation

The sixth, seventh and eighth stages of the path are: *Dharana*, *Dhyana* and *Samadhi*. The first includes methods of concentration which focus the mind on a single point. The second leads to a state of stillness and detachment in which the mind is centered, but open to the universe. In the third, *Samadhi*, the mind has expanded to become universal and the joy of oneness is experienced. The Buddha practiced these three but added *Bhakti*, or worship, and *Karma*, or service. In unison, these five lead to that state of religious ecstasy called Enlightenment. The Buddha reached Enlightenment through Yoga, became free, and began to teach others the Way.

Buddhism has three main forms: the *Hinayana*, or narrow way, the *Mahayana*, or broad way and the Tantric, or esoteric, form. In Japan there are very many Buddhist sects representing all these main forms in a variety of ways. All of them are derived from the original teaching of the Buddha, who taught a nuclear idea of immense potential. Subsequently each founder of a sect took only what he could grasp. Each sect has its own interpretation of the original teaching, its own sacred writings, and its own methods of training. Whilst the Buddha's teaching applies to all possible situations in life, the sectarian teachings, being partial, necessarily cannot. Of course, the men who founded sects had exceptional talents, but the sects only prospered according to who ruled Japan at the time and which teaching was popular with them. Usually, this association with power led the sects into moral corruption and spiritual degeneracy. Indeed, we can see that religions generally have never been spiritually creative when they have depended upon the written word, ignoring practice and spiritual experience. When Christianity arrived in Rome, it was fresh, vivid, and full of spiritual vitality. Christians would not give up their spiritual beliefs even when faced with a martyr's death. Many felt so inspired and full of enthusiasm that they deliberately sought such an end. But this white-hot heat of faith could not be indefinitely maintained and, by the 12th Century A.D., when Thomas Aquinas was writing his theology, the Church ruled the world and had become thoroughly corrupted. An account of the Church of those days is found in the contemporary novel *Decameron*.

Another example is afforded by early Ch'an Buddhism in China. Northern Ch'an became, for a time, the orthodox religion of the state and was soon corrupted. Southern Ch'an, which was called Zen in Japan, was never politically powerful and yet continued to produce spiritual genius and a succession of great teachers. This is apparently a basic law, that there are recurrent cycles of creativity and degeneration in religion. Spirituality cannot survive the association with worldly power and wealth. Conversely, folk religion, which has almost always been associated with poverty, retains its vitality and purity. It was the folk religion of the Heian Period in Japan, for example, which generated the spiritual vitality of the succeeding Kamakura Period. This was the time when Zen became popular in Japan. At all times there have been poor men who have risen to positions of power and authority simply because of their truth and piety. They were men who lived close to nature and were not interested in wearing the glittering robes of religion. Such men provide the force which generates history because they understand the value of practical experience and can catch the essence of truth amidst the welter of irrelevance.

There is a Japanese saying—"Those who live in luxury will surely fall." We should never waste our sympathy on those who lose their power and position through laziness and pride. Those who manage to cling on to high places and prestige in spite of soft living are actually worse. The vital point is that power and wealth corrupt and that the only sure road to knowledge is through practical involvement. It is through practical experience alone that we can create our own personalities and become real individuals. Reject luxury, never try to impress others, devote yourself fully to your purpose, and you will live according to the laws of nature. These principles can also be applied to religion to ensure that it is not swallowed by power and made authoritarian and narrow. True religion should teach people how to be, how to live rightly, and how to actualize their full potential. The religion which is supremely fitted to do this is Yogic Buddhism. It was only after twenty years of study and thought that I realized this and began my life of seeking truth through Yoga. In the course of that search, I have been initiated into many religions and practiced many kinds of health regimes. I am thankful for this experience but without the help of God I would never have begun the search. Without the many experiences of joy and suffering which have come to me through my good *karmic* relationships, I would never have gained my present understanding of life.

I have faced death many times, especially during the war when I worked as a secret agent for my country, and later, too, when I developed intestinal cancer. Out of these experiences, I have come to know the love of God and the real meaning of faith. If we had no difficulties to face and overcome, we would never be moved to ask the important questions about life and death. We would never begin to seek the truth. This process is the only way to discover and cultivate yourself and, for purposes of explanation, it can be analyzed into three phases. First comes physical training and practical experience. Secondly, study and reflection to develop spiritual and moral sensitivity. Thirdly, the application of the knowledge thus gained to practical life situations. This process, constantly repeated, changes knowledge into wisdom so that we can acquire a true understanding of life through our own efforts.

Each of us has been given many *karmic* relationships with other people and our interactions with them are vital teachings for us. The attitude of faith enables us to receive and use these teachings creatively and to see them as expressions of God's love. Through this experience we develop our highest potential and become of the greatest service to others and to society. Yoga taught me this holistic view and gave me the method of teaching it to people. Yoga combines all methods and can be entered from any "direction," so that all your previous experience of life is of value. Yoga has helped me to become really free, for it is the only practical way to raise the level of consciousness to the divine.

The Yogic method enables us to carry out a continuous objective examination of our life experience by suspending our habit of making value judgments. In this way we avoid mental conflict as well as all forms of attachment so that we can naturally generate a thirst for the truth. The Buddha is our greatest exemplar and there is no other religion besides his Yogic Buddhism which can enable us to reach Enlightenment. Although the three last stages of the Yogic path seem similar, the content of each is quite different. The way to freedom is to understand and practice them all. People usually assume that there are many preparations to be made before entering *samyama*, but the method of Yoga is simple and clear. Through the three phases of practice, reflection and application, which I have described, we become more and more human, developing both our inner life and our social relationships.

Unlike sectarian religious teachings, Yoga can be applied to every situation we meet in life and suits all historical periods. Only in Yoga, is found the complete unification of practice and learning. Neither of these two is sufficient alone. We need both in order to accurately assess information and work out the way to apply the teachings of Yoga in our own lives. If we want to hear the voice of inner wisdom, we have to unify knowledge and experience, mind and body, and try to be detached and free. This aim must be consistently pursued in our daily lives and in every situation. The more we can broaden and deepen our practice, the more open will our minds become and the nearer we will be to perfect freedom and oneness in *satori*. The Yogin is one who conducts his own religion, formulates his own truth through experience, and relies on no-one. Only that is the true, eternal religion which knows no limitations.

In the Orient, there is an ancient saying—"He who speaks does not know, and he who knows does not speak." This perfectly exemplifies the way of Yoga. Yoga has developed for several thousands of years without benefit of sacred writings and yet it has come down to us as a living religion. There are two attitudes possible in religion: the practical one of the esoteric sects and the more theoretical one of the exoteric sects which look to their sacred writings for inspiration. Yet, the fact is that the founders of religions and of the religious sects were all men of an extremely practical bent. It is only their followers who later abandoned the way of practice. In Japan, we find this practical religion in the esoteric *Shingon* sect. To this day, the *Shingon* believer goes on a pilgrimage around a circuit of eighty-eight temples. This is a very practical training which strengthens the body and purifies the mind. Both the *Shingon* and the *Tendai* sects maintain their own training Dōjōs and give practical teaching, according to their sutras, which includes fasting.

The word "*Shingon*" combines the syllables "shin," meaning "truth" and "gon," meaning "words"—a *Shingon* is thus a *mantra*. By repetition of the *mantra*, mind and body are unified and brought to oneness with the truth. When I was staying at a Buddhist temple in Tibet, I found that they also made use of *mantras* and that this was only one hint of the connection between Tibetan Buddhism and *Shingon*. Both also embody the teaching of *sanmitsu*, for example, the use of *mantra* to bring about the integration of body, speech and mind. Kūkai, the founder of *Shingon*, brought the *mantra* method from China to Japan along with many valuable sutras. *Shingon* has taken much from Yoga and from Tibet, where references to a *Yuga* sect can be found in ancient Buddhist sutras. In Japan, there is a mountain called *Yuga* and the word *Yoga* often appears in the small *Shingon* shrines which are found all over the country. It is, however, difficult to know exactly what kind of Yoga is implied for there do not appear to be any sutras which describe the Yoga practices of *Shingon*. We can be sure that there have always been those people who gave all their attention to physical and mental discipline but, at the present time, such training forms only a small, but important, part of the activity of these esoteric sects.

Kūkai himself was an extremely active and practical person. When he was young, he undertook much rigorous ascetic training and, later, established a training center on Mount Koya. His irrigation works in Shikoku, the southern island of Japan, still survive as a testimony to his untiring service to the community. He also founded the first Japanese university. Kūkai was both a practical man and a religious genius.

It is because Yoga is a religion of direct, practical experience that it is eternally renewed and always possesses the characteristics of a new religion. Many religious teachers in India, Central Asia, and the Middle East told me that they recognized that Yoga is the Mother of all religions and teaches the essence of the Way to Enlightenment. Yoga in India today is, however, very far from being real Yoga. Yoga must be a complete life-style, a way of self-cultivation and genuinely lead us to true meditation. Those who have experienced meditation training at the Okidō Dōjō are surprised to find that it is full of vitality. In concentration sitting practice they find that the physical demands of meditation often make the beginner sweat copiously. It is almost like having a sauna bath. Later, the mind and body become very relaxed and tranquil. When tension and relaxation are balanced, real meditation can begin. This training brings also a new quality to movement, so that, even in the midst of violent activity, we experience the utmost calm. When I walk amongst my students as they meditate, I am filled with tremendous vitality, or *prana*. Treading silently, I correct only those whose posture and expression tells me that they are trying to do their very best. Those who are dull and listless are ignored and this lack of attention stimulates them to try harder. Gradually they all become silent and calm and their breath becomes deep and long. Those who have participated in our meditation realize that this is the real training. Restlessness and fear are overcome; neurosis and sickness disappear almost irrespective of the student's attitude.

2. The Real Meaning of Unification and Detachment

When the body's power, concentrated in the *Hara*, and the mind's power, concentrated in the sixth *Chakra*, or "third eye," are brought together, this is unification. It is to become centered and natural and to return to the original condition of body and mind. In this state, body and mind cooperate harmoniously to perform the work of life and this is Yoga. The essential principle of training is to do all actions consciously and with full attention. In other words, with real awareness. The Life-Force is a manifestation of

The Real Meaning of Unification and Detachment / 87

God, so that having unified body and mind, the next step is to become unified with the Divine.

Body and mind are integrated through action; it is the three stage process of Yoga consciously performed, as previously described. When reading a book, for example, we should also engage the body in the task by being aware of posture as well as mentally concentrating. Reading is thus transformed into a training and, further, we must study how to make practical use of what we learn whilst reading in our daily life. Another example is provided by the common example of carrying things. We should carry things with awareness of our actions and also with awareness of the value of material goods. Then we can experience gratitude to all those whose work has produced these things. If it is so, materials will be well cared for and not wasted. Human life will be truly human and naturally dignified.

Total Unification is Yoga: Although most teachings have the merit of containing some truth, they are thereby characterized by a basic imbalance. We cannot gain real Enlightenment through systems that deal only with the body, or only with the mind, for they are like a bird with only one wing. A balanced way must integrate the development of body and mind and give the most benefit to family life, society, and nature. In Japanese, a Dō means "a complete way of life," and Okidō aims at the realization of the ideal life through practical Dōjō training. For this reason, Okidō is real Yoga which seeks complete balance and harmony. It has taken me more than thirty years of study and practice to discover these principles and incorporate them into one logical system. Yoga inspired me to give expression to the philosophy of totality and the religion of wholeness in a practical way. In a very real sense, therefore, I am just a beginner! Yoga means the natural condition of coexistence and coprosperity of all forms of life and I always try to apply this principle consistently. When translated into English, the name of the Mishima Dōjō means—"The Yoga Training Dōjō For The Benefit Of All Life." The clear difference between present day Indian Yoga and Okidō is this: Indian Yoga is no longer fully integrated into the fabric of social life.

To do everything in a centered condition is the fundamental rule of training. If we are physically centered in the *Hara* and mentally centered with the mind of worship and service, we have maximum stamina. We must always do things totally, even in physical exercise and, for example, when running we should run not only forwards, but also backwards and sideways. I call this principle "the stamina method." At first it is difficult to do everything with complete mental and physical willingness. By continual daily training and the practice of detachment we can learn to do everything gladly without the slightest reluctance. In its perfection, this state of mind is called *Mushin*: it is the mind of Emptiness which is the aim of Zen. *Mushin* is a significant step towards *satori*; that state of total love and oneness in which we naturally love even our enemies. In their different ways, the Buddha and the Christ both epitomized this state of being in their lives.

Our daily lives are without real value unless we regard them as the training ground for *satori*. Yoga bids us to use every life situation to complete ourselves and to serve others. A narrowly intellectual understanding of the meaning of love is far from being sufficient. Living in this total way enables us to distil the essence of culture and knowledge from our heritage and to gain a profound communication with life. It also allows us to make the maximum contribution to the human race and to the entire living universe. Through dedicating our lives in this way, we make ourselves worthy, noble and dignified. It is a way which bridges science, philosophy and religion and is generated by the apparently simple three-fold method of training, reflection and application which is taught by Yoga. The greatest exponent of this way was the Buddha and this entire book is really a tribute to his magnificent example.

Live fully, harmoniously and well: In their normal state, the body and mind of human beings are far from unified. Consequently, they develop the symptoms of disunity: neurosis and illness. How can we transcend this state and reach *Mushin*? The simple answer is, by doing everything with full, conscious awareness of what we are do-

The Real Meaning of Unification and Detachment / 89

ing, and why. When an action is performed in this positive, active manner, the simple things of daily life become the objects of our meditation. When all actions are done perfectly in this way you will already be living in the state of *satori*. Yet it is actually nothing more than having full respect for yourself and others.

Sometimes people tell me that they have become weak through lack of exercise, but if so, it is quite needless. Although I spend a large proportion of my time in my study, I manage to maintain my physical condition and muscle tone unimpaired. The reason is simply that I do everything, especially reading and writing, with my total body and mind. To use ourselves in this way is true seriousness. We say that a person who works in this way is doing things with his heart and soul. Deep interest in a task automatically unifies the body and mind and this principle can, and should, be applied to everything in life. For example, when people eat they normally think only of eating and the mind tends to be occupied with thoughts about not eating what they dislike. When people are restless, they think only of their restlessness. The point is that they can unify the body and mind only too easily in a negative direction. The crux of the problem of body-mind unification is thus only to change the direction of the will towards positive and creative things. The ability to do this is generated by our daily Yoga training. In life we must first decide which things are good for us and, having decided, devote ourselves totally to mastering them. The best way is to apply the three-fold Yogic method of training, reflection and application to whatever we decide to do.

Consciousness is unified in the cerebral cortex by means of concentration and physical power is unified in the *Hara* through the breath. That there is a close connection between these two is easily proved. If you concentrate strength in the *Hara* by correct breathing, you will notice that the mind becomes clear and calm as well as physical power being increased. When we do things in a *Hara*-centered state, we can feel that the nerves, hormones and muscles are balanced and that emotions and desires are stable. When body and mind are in good condition, we can easily unify them and give ourselves totally to any task. When they are not in good condition, this is difficult. We have to learn to make situations which will help us to achieve this unification. Teaching others, or demonstrating our skill and ability to others are situations which stimulate us to make our best efforts. By putting ourselves in difficult situations we can most quickly improve our ability.

When we do things in a centered and balanced way, we soon find the best methods to employ. This is the first stage in which body, mind and technique become one. In the second stage of learning we must train our minds to the task of discovering the most sophisticated techniques. In the third stage, we have to incorporate the higher skills into our practice until they become effortless. The fourth and final stage, when all our learning, techniques, and practice are the natural expression of the unified body and mind, is called Enlightenment.

3. Dharana: The Sixth Stage

(1) The meaning of concentration

Dharana is the second stage of Zen discipline and means to unify the power of body and mind through concentration. *Pratyahara* is the first stage. *Dharana* means to consolidate consciousness by making the mind one-pointed. The stage after *Dharana* is *Dhyana* and this depends upon having condensed the power of body and mind in the earlier stage. *Dharana* is essentially a Yang exercise consisting of the discipline of the breath and concentration of power. *Dhyana* is the complimentary Yin phase of release. In the Yang phase, tension is created and power is compacted. In the Yin phase, body and mind are expanded and given controlled release.

After achieving this balance of maximum Yin and Yang power, the mind becomes empty of limitations and enters into *satori*. In the unifying exercise of *Dharana*, the conscious objective is to make all aspects of consciousness accessible, or to unify consciousness and unconsciousness. For this purpose we must first unify the body and, then, integrate body and mind by means of the harmonized breath.

The principle training is to learn to do everything with the whole body and mind without a shade of reluctance. This state of totally one-pointed power is known in Japanese as *Nenriki* and it can give rise to supernormal powers, such as telekinesis. *Nenriki* is actually the most rational and efficient way of using power and enables you to express your ability fully. The more one-pointedly power can be applied the more effective it will be.

(2)   Three kinds of concentration

In *Shingon* consciousness is unified by means of *mantra*; in *Soto* Zen, by sitting; and in *Rinzai* Zen by the use of the *Koan*. I have tried all these ways and many others, but found that they all involved great difficulty. By contrast, the way of unification of Yoga is understandable and easy even for beginners and children. This is the broad way to *satori*.

The right way to attain unification of consciousness depends upon personality; each person can find the way which is best for himself. Broadly speaking, there are three methods, as follows:

(a) Conscious *Dharana* by means of the various practices which will be decribed in the later part of this chapter.
(b) Unconscious *Dharana* which is the result of *karmic* inheritance. A great musician, for example, has gained unification in this way.
(c) The *Dharana* of attachment. The ability to play like a child induces concentration, but since it depends upon attachment, we become unaware of others. Releasing our attention from the object is difficult, so that it is really a form of bondage.

The only worthwhile way of unifying consciousness is one in which we can release ourselves freely from the object of our attention. For the vast majority of people, the methods included under (a) above are the most practical.

(3) Make good use of suffering and worldly attachment

Suffering is the absence of unity, for a mind which is conditioned is in a disunified state and becomes attached to, or dependent upon, this or that psychological crutch. The mind is subservient to a continuous stream of thoughts, which are often random and aimless, so that concentration is very difficult. For a long time I saw this state of mind only negatively as a hindrance to concentration and a barrier which would prevent me from developing that clear bright mind which does not become attached and is free from the domination of the contents of consciousness.

Yoga gave me the hint which led to the solution of this problem. Once you decide that you will worry consciously and thoroughly to the bitter end, that you will become the suffering, then it becomes a training in concentration and you pass through and beyond the suffering. This demonstrates to us that worldly thought has little power to disturb the mind which is detached, equanimous and free. For example, if dirty water is poured into a vessel and left to stand, the dirt will settle to the bottom after a time. Meditation is like this for the practice of non-attachment is like leaving the water to stand. *Mushin* mind does not mean that thought ceases but that, through detachment, thoughts which arise are allowed also to sink. So although there are many thoughts, it is the same as if there were none for the mind is untroubled by them.

The physiological effect of concentration is that the sympathetic nervous system is stimulated. Although it gives the impression that you like to be serious and severe, concentration is practiced to gain peace and serenity. A calm mind results when the sympathetic nervous system energizes the parasympathetic nervous system and a balance is achieved. When this occurs there is great stability and you can enter into *Mushin*. This process works according to the principle of balance maintenance. The negative will always call forth the positive so that repression will intensify desire because any phenomenon naturally attracts its opposite.

Any meditation system which lacks *Kinen* is unbalanced. This is true of *Zazen* taught in the Zen temples and the meditation of Indian

Yoga. The former lacks relaxation whilst the latter lacks tension. The key to obtaining a true balance of dynamic and static power is the practice of concentration concurrently with discipline of the breath. After you have built up concentration it is essential to release it. The way to release it is not to revert to the worldly mind but to go beyond concentration to *Mushin*. In that state, total attention is naturally given to each and every activity, so that the mind seems to become the eye, or the ear, and each sense is unbelievably heightened. It is sometimes described as the condition of *Happomoku*; of being able to see and feel in all directions at once. It is a very useful condition for the warrior.

From *Isshin*, or concentration, we reach to *Mushin*.

(4) Hara power

The effect of *Dharana* is mainly to bring power to the more stable parts of the body. If you consciously breath abdominally, power will condense in the *Hara* and you will be strong in the lower abdomen, legs, and waist. Also the tension will be released from the upper parts and the body will be natural; that is: the head will be Yin and cold, the lower parts Yang and hot. When this physiological condition is present, the sympathetic nervous system works better and a hormone is released which activates the parasympathetic nervous system and produces a sense of calmness. The production of adrenalin, which arouses and excites the body, is naturally balanced. Without *Hara* power, energy flows to the upper part of the body, the breath becomes shallow, adrenalin is released, and only the sympathetic nervous system is stimulated. There is thus a lack of balance and the acid content of the blood becomes high. From long experience I can definitely say that the majority of illnesses would be prevented if *Hara* power was present.

When there is good *Hara* power, the breath becomes deep and well-adjusted. The muscles of the abdomen are flexible and spread widely so that every breath is strong. The diaphragm has maximum freedom to move up and down and the chest is fully expanded. In this condition the whole body is breathing and you feel that the upper part is firmly supported by the lower part.

Amongst all the parts of the body, it is the lower abdomen where breath and body fluids are most liable to stagnate. This causes bad blood circulation and tiredness of mind. When the abdomen is free to move largely and strongly, the blood is not able to stagnate and circulation to the brain is also increased. When abdominal breathing becomes habitual, the abdominal muscles are naturally strengthened. The center of gravity of the body is lowered and all actions are naturally performed from the *Hara*. If the sympathetic nervous system is working well and abdominal breathing is habitual, even the effect of a tremendous shock or surprise subsides quickly and all actions are performed with a clear bright, mind. When a person has good *Hara*, he is always able to preserve balance and harmony.

The power of *Hara* has a close connection with the mental attitude of willingness, or positive mind. If you feel curious, or take a deep interest in a task, the body and mind are full of power. The *Hara* is strong and consciousness becomes clear. That is why we have good *Hara* and great power in times of danger, or when hovering between life and death. I have already explained that laughter promotes good *Hara*. If you devote yourself to any activity with pleasure, laughter and willingness, things always go well. You can fully express your ability and all your activities become healthy exercise. Sometimes people die shortly after retirement. The reason is that they have lost the activity which they took most interest in and no longer do the things which raised *Hara* power. They lose physical balance, breath balance and the balance of mind.

(5) To act and understand with Hara

Human beings need *Hara* because *Hara* means that you do not become obsessed. You can do anything with full concentration but also drop it instantly if need be. To indulge in things is dangerous; it is attachment rather than love. The Buddha said "Meet neither the one you love nor the one you hate." If we love a person too much we cannot live without them and if we hate too much we are also emotionally conditioned. So we should try to avoid these extremes of feeling, just as we should try to avoid attachment to possessions.

Theoretically this seems to contradict the concept of love, but concepts do frequently contradict practical wisdom. This only demonstrates the artificiality of conceptualization. True love means that there is a sense of oneness with everyone and not just a specific individual. This is the perfect cooperation of *Atman* and *Brahman* in Yoga.

(6) Mind and Hara

When there is intense concentration, *Hara* power is needed to balance the high electrical potential of the brain. There are often spontaneous corrections of energy build-up in the body such as a fit of coughing which disperses tension in the chest and shoulders. One of the chief effects of Chinese acupuncture is to neutralize or recirculate the electrical potential in the body. When concentration of consciousness increases the electrical potential of the brain you should avoid putting power into the hands, neck or shoulders. The optimum state of the body-mind for meditation is attained when the energy potential in the lower body balances that of the mind. Additionally the focussing of physical energy in the *Hara* center releases tension from the upper part of the body. In that state you can take in sufficient oxygen for the brain. The brain needs more than two hundred times as much oxygen, cell for cell, as other parts of the body.

The brain has three main layers. The intellect, or rationality, is a function of the topmost layer, or cerebral cortex. Physiology and instinctive reactions are controlled by the next deeper layer, the midbrain. The basic instincts and deep emotions arise from the most primitive layer, known as the hindbrain. At best, these three work in perfect accord but sometimes become disunified. In extreme cases, one layer becomes dormant and the other two almost cease to function.

Of these three layers, the mid-brain is the strongest in the majority of people, so that they are over-affected by their emotional reactions to conditions and situations. Animals, too, are deeply affected by their feelings and can sense the emotional climate instantly. It is the hindbrain which generates association of ideas and gives rise to fantasy, but the cerebral cortex adds to these mental constructions. What comes from the hindbrain is initially stronger than what comes from the cerebral cortex, but when rationality is developed the latter can control the former. Usually however, the instincts do not follow the dictates of the mind. The decisive factor is often the mid-brain, for if it reinforces the instincts, the person will yield to temptation. Strange, abnormal, or childish actions are the result. People in this condition are carried away by the impulse of the moment and often become neurotic or commit criminal acts.

Theoretically, the way to mental health is to develop rationality enough to control the deeper layers. This is not so easy, however, as these older layers are very strong and can easily by-pass the power of reason. The more Yin the condition of the head and the stronger and more stable rationality can become. The entire autonomic nervous system become more powerful. There is a way of ensuring the harmonious cooperation of all three levels which utilizes this fact. If you have strong *Hara*, the flood of emotions from the hindbrain is calmed. The autonomous nervous system also becomes calm. The autonomous nervous system becomes balanced and stable and instinctual appetites are minimized.

Human beings are apt to become excited and tense very easily under the conditions of modern life. Specific training in relaxation and release becomes necessary to regain the natural condition of harmony. The effect of a developed consciousness and walking erect with a vertical spine has been to lessen our ability to control the instincts. Other factors which have contributed to this problem are that natural abdominal breathing has been forgotten, the waist and abdomen have become weak, and there is too much acid in the blood due to over-eating. If we work to correct these factors our ability to relax and to control instincts will be increased.

When you raise *Hara* power through *Danshari*, *Shusei*, and *Meiso*, you can easily live on little food and control the deep instinctual desires. Such training stimulates the highest human potential. The ability to extract the utmost nourishment from food is increased, the heat of the stomach and coolness of the head is improved and, even though it becomes very strong, you can control desire. The efficiency and power of every organ is raised. When the influence of the hindbrain is controlled, the higher levels of consciousness will more easily direct all our activities. Even those habits which have been ingrained since birth will be subject to the power of reason and the whole of your life will become sacred.

(7) Memory and heredity

When we want to memorize something it is common practice to write it down or repeat it frequently in a loud voice. Sheer intellectual ability is fine for solving problems but does not help us to memorize information. The work of memorizing is performed by the hindbrain. Another way of memorizing is to experience things with the whole body and mind. For example, the body can memorize the feeling of the word "disgust" and this can be associated with the spelling and pronunciation. Similarly, anyone learning English can remember the word "beautiful" by associating it with the memory of some beautiful object, such as a lily. Repeating information from memory reinforces the ability to recall the new information which flows out and makes it a conditioned reflex. Actually, when we do this, we are processing information coming from the hindbrain through the cerebral cortex. In consequence, most mnemonics, or aids to memory, are calculated to impress the deeper levels of consciousness handled by the hindbrain.

Some of the more common methods of memorizing are:

(a) Repeating with concentration.
(b) Making the information to be memorized into a game.
(c) By means of a sudden shock, or vivid impression.
(d) Sleeping after reading.

It is generally acknowledged that memories are acquired after birth and are not inherited. We can't hand on knowledge, but a part of memory may affect the character of our descendants through genetic transmission of cell structures. Such a "memory" is not knowledge. The evolutionary changes in living species occur by means of mutation, and natural selection. The experience of individuals after birth is a powerful factor in this process. Strength and wisdom help to preserve the species and promote cooperation with the process of necessary change. We relate to our ancestors through our genetic inheritance as well as through civilization and culture. The cooperation of many factors and many people has contributed to the life of every individual alive today. This "effort of life" affects the subsequent generations. We are the fruits of this effort on the part of our ancestors and will hand on our inheritance, adding to it our own contribution. It is simply the practice of natural gratitude to try to develop oneself for the better. What is handed down are the basic attitudes to life which have become conditioned reflexes or instinctual urges. As children we receive this natural heritage, but we must strive to improve and refine what we receive as well as add to it. To do this we have to strengthen our power of rationality and build positive habits and attitudes into the lower levels of consciousness. The first step is to create a good character and an instinctive liking for the ideal Yogic way of life. This leads us to the unification of the various levels of thought.

When we associate with others we should try to discern which part of the brain is dominant. If a girl says, "I feel cold" she may mean, "lets light the stove," if it is the higher level of the brain which is in control. If the middle level is dominant she could mean, "embrace me" or, if the thought comes from the lower level, "I want a new overcoat." We can judge which level a person is tuned into from several factors. If the eyes are bright and intelligent looking, the voice animated, and the posture upright and stable, the cerebral cortex is in control. If the impulse comes from the mid-brain, tension will be released from the body and the chin will tend to drop. When the hindbrain controls the posture will be slouched and the chin raised. The eyes may show grief or other deep emotion. All strong feelings have their natural postures too. Couples in love tend to sit close together and bend forwards, for their feelings come from the deep levels of consciousness. So too, if a girl is thinking of a loved one whilst sitting at a table or desk, she will tend to lean forward and support her chin with both hands. It is a common place experience that women, especially, do not immediately express their real attitude. They will often say "no" when they mean "yes" because rationality does not instantly interpret what is coming from the deeper levels of consciousness. Sometimes a woman will ask her husband to take her for a day out. She may mean only that she wants to see new sights, or wish to indicate that she requires affection, or just the excitement of buying something new. If you can control yourself and observe acutely, you can know the minds of others and hence know what to say to them. Every teacher should be a person with good *Hara* and self control for this reason. The Buddha was the greatest teacher the world has ever known precisely because of his immense self-control and acute perception.

(8) The practice of Dharana

Unity of consciousness, or concentration, is not the end of our development but an essential intermediate step. Concentration is favorable for further progress, but the body and mind also require relaxation, rest and sleep. Although we may obtain a little *Hara* power, we cannot have a developed *Hara* without sustained practice of *Meiso Yoga* for at least one year.

Warming-up: Before *Dharana* it is necessary to prepare yourself, just as a baseball player warms up with catchball, or a Martial Artist does *Katas*. Such preparation should be neither too hard nor too strong. Before concentration it is good to sing a song which disposes the mind towards spiritual things, or to do breathing exercises. Some people like to play a musical instrument, such as the *Shakuhachi*. Before doing any exercise it is best to relax, then breath in and put power into appropriate areas of the body. Following this we should do a breath retention, or *kumbhaka*, and afterwards, exhale and release power. At the same time the visualization of *prana*, or *ki*, is a good practice.

Meditation practice has three phases:

(a) *Choshinho* —The way of adjusting posture.
(b) *Chosokuho* —The way of adjusting breath.
(c) *Mushinho* —The way of empty mind.

This is an analytical division from a different aspect to that which is expressed as *Dharana, Dhyana* and *Samadhi*. Both possesses a certain lack of precision and artificiality in practice.

Choshinho: This is the practice of a stable sitting position. There are many variants, but the following two are best for most people. The pose of the adept involves sitting with legs crossed and one foot resting on top of the other. Easy pose is likewise a folded leg posture, but both feet rest on the floor with one in front of the other. The leg which is most difficult to bend should be placed to the rear.

Adopt the pose of your choice, stretch the waist, raise and spread the chest and leave the eyes open. Raise the upper arms slightly so that an egg could be inserted under the armpits. Pull in the chin and release tension from the neck and shoulders. Stretch the abdominal muscles upwards and downwards, tighten the anal sphincter muscle slightly, and concentrate your power in the *Hara*. At first you will find this posture difficult, but it will become natural after a few weeks of regular daily practice. *Yogasanas* and Okidō corrective exercises help to make the body supple, so that sitting becomes easy. Essentially, the chest must be spread and the tension released from the upper body and the solar plexus. The shoulders should be relaxed and dropped and you will feel the supporting power of the lower abdominal muscle taking over.

Chosokuho: At first we have to practice right breathing consciously, but if we persevere the breathing will become rhythmical and the muscular action will be more unified. A quiet, deep breath is normal in whole body breathing. When a person is entering into the condition of *satori* the breath naturally becomes longer and more peaceful.

Mushinho: This is the practice of the empty mind which is mental release. At first we concentrate upon one specific thing but, later, awareness of this object disappears. *Mushin* is the condition of being nothing, yet paradoxically, everything. Now concentration is effortless, yet not focused onto any one object. It is wide, peaceful and universal. This change is not brought about deliberately but occurs naturally when all the conditions are right. Because of this we cannot say exactly where *Dharana* ends and *Dhyana* begins. The same kind of situation exists as in the continuous interplay between change, balance, and stability in the movement of a living being. Because it is a dynamic state, none of these factors ever exists in isolation. Nonetheless, they are real factors. So, too, are *Dharana* and *Dhyana*.

The Concentration of Consciousness: There are many practices for increasing the power of concentration. Counting the breaths, focussing upon a Zen *koan*—which is an insoluble question—concentrating on the *Hara*, or on the inner sounds of the body are some of the more usual methods. In Yoga the following ways have been traditionally recognized:

(a) *Dakurita:* Concentration on the sixth *Chakra*, the space between the eyes.
(b) *Nashikagura Dharishita:* Concentration on the tip of the nose. This way is used in Zen.
(c) *Anahata Tanani:* Concentration on the inner sounds of the body. The main sounds of the heart are said to be *Aa, Na, Ha,* and *Ta,* hence *Anahata,* but there are many others. To turn the attention within, *Shambhava Mudra* is used. Both hands are employed to close the eyes, ears, nose and mouth.
(d) *Mantra:* Concentration on a word or phrase in order to unify consciousness. The best example is the great *mantra Aum,* which is repeated aloud or silently. There are many *mantras* within

the Japanese religious tradition also. The *Nembutsu* and the *Daimoku* are both very popular. *Mantras* are also found in other religions, such as Islam and Taoism.

In *Aum*, the sound "A" is opening. Lean backwards slightly and spread the chest. "A" releases the power from the hands, puts power in the abdomen and makes the body cool and the blood alkaline. When a dog is happy, he also barks with joyous "A" sounds and stands with his legs open. When a person is injured he says "Ah" because this cools the body and helps to relieve tension. When a person is pleased to see you, "A" sounds will predominate in his speech. The released body condition corresponds to happiness and the tight one to misery.

The sound "O" is made with a round mouth. Lean slightly forwards to make the body tight and to stretch the back muscles. "O" puts power into the chest and prevents the release of heat from the body. We say "O" naturally when we step into a cold bath. "O" puts power into the hands and makes the blood acid. A dog in distress makes "O" whining sounds and barks with a "rounded" bark.

The sound "UM" is a closing sound. It makes the shoulders relaxed and so the power can flow down to the *Hara*. The effect on the blood is to balance the acid and alkaline content and make it neutral. This sound intensifies the power of body and mind and unifies them together.

(e) *Shata Ataru:* In this method we begin by concentrating on the breath and then change to one of the *Chakras* when concentration deepens. In *Theravada* Buddhism, it is usual to change to the third *Chakra*, the *Hara*, or the sixth, between the eyes. Such a change merely follows the practice in *Yogasanas* of changing concentration from one part of the body to another. So too, in attaining *satori*, it is easier at first to concentrate on one specific thing but, afterwards, in *Mushin*, the object of meditation constantly changes with the flux of reality. In *Kundalini* Yoga, consciousness is concentrated firstly at the base of the spine, but is then moved progressively upwards to include all the *Chakras*. The aim is to unify the individual life with the Divine. It is the union of *Atman* and *Brahman* attained by using the basic sexual energy of the body as the medium.

(f) *Bhakti Yoga:* Here the mind is brought to union with God through the power of faith. Attention is concentrated solely on the beloved teacher, or the Divine Lord. The object of love brings the mind to one-pointedness through intense devotion.

(g) *Karma Yoga:* The whole of the life of the *Karma* Yogin is concentrated upon serving others. Self is sacrificed in the service of mankind. The greatest *Karma* Yogin of modern times was undoubtedly Mahatma Gandhi.

4. The Seventh Stage

(1) The Dhyqna of Yoga and Zen

The three stages of *Samyama* are practiced one after the other and all together, as I explained previously. Although *Dharana* and *Dhyana* appear to be similar, their opposite extremes are actually quite different. Where *Dharana* is one-pointed concentration, fixed and unmoving, *Dhyana* is the universal mind, ever flowing with life and so empty of all limitation. At the physical level, *Dharana* is contraction and integration, whilst *Dhyana* is expansion and release. In the Yang state of *Dharana* you feel powerful and stimulated, whilst in the Yin state of *Dhyana*, you feel quiet, peaceful and refreshed. But peace does not mean a condition in which energy is released and the body is in a state of total collapse. Energy is full but it is balanced with relaxation; the body is static and consciousness is very clear. *Dhyana* is the meditation of the Buddha, but it has undergone changes in the course of being transmitted from India, via China to Japan. In China, the word *Dharana* became Ch'an and, in Japan, Zen.

If you continue to practice *Dharana* it will lead you to *Dhyana*. Everyone can attain *Dharana* and *Dhyana*, if they practice sufficiently, regardless of their background, experience or religion. *Dhyqna* produces a stable mental condition in which the mind will not fall into confusion, even though you are faced with a naked sword, are perilously hanging from a cliff, or are attacked by a ferocious wild animal. In the past, meditation training included many dangers, such as sitting beneath a sword which would fall and kill you if you failed to maintain correct posture. The training systems of all religions formerly sought to make knowing and doing one, but they have nowadays become imbalanced. Okidō teaches, by less extreme methods, that knowing and doing, mind and body, are one. This is done by insisting that everyone must participate fully, without reluctance, in a well-rounded training, which avoids narrow specialization.

(2) How to practice Dhyana

In *Dhyana*, the eyes may be closed, half-open, or fully open and, in *Meiso Yoga*, we use the fully open position. First of all, use appropriate cushions and sit in one of the recognized postures of meditation: full lotus, half-lotus, or the Japanese kneeling position, called *Seiza*.

(a) Pull in the chin and stretch the spine upwards. Imagine that the eyeballs are being pulled into the head and also that you are being drawn upwards by means of a string attached to the crown of the head. If the chin is raised, the spine is bent, the eyeballs tend to relax and the eyeballs protrude.
(b) Spread your chest to right and left so that the upper part of the body becomes relaxed.
(c) Push the waist forward and stretch the abdominal muscles upwards and downwards. Think of the hips going down and feel energy flowing into the lower half of the body. Touch the tongue to the roof of the mouth and hold the lips slightly tensed. Tighten the anal sphincter muscle by slightly drawing in the abdomen. Finally, put slight tension into your inner thighs to bring power to the center of balance, the *Hara*. In this condition, the mind as well as the *Hara* is energized and the resistance to all kinds of poison is remarkably increased.

The Seventh Stage / 105

The optimum physical condition is that in which all energies and functions consuming and expelling, tension and relaxation, Yin and Yang are developed to their maximum potential and then brought to a state of balance and integration. The spine, for example, is the most Yang part of the body and the muscles the most Yin. When the spine is fully charged with energy the muscles can be relaxed. A regime of diet, exercise, and training of the breath, balance, and mind is necessary to bring the body to its full power. Further, two attitudes to life are possible: the first is the normal one of doing your best out of self-interest; the second is to relinquish all desire for reward. I will not waste time on considering totally negative attitudes.

A good way of becoming physically centered is to make the mental resolve to release tension in the various parts of the body until deep relaxation is achieved. In all activities, we should try to combine right posture, right breathing, and right mental attitude. This the principle of *sanmitsu*, three ways in one, which can be effectively applied to many things. The general rule is that the remaining two factors cannot attain optimum development if the first one is incorrect. If the first one is corrected, the others will automatically become right. In the case of posture, breathing and mental attitude, the best way is for the beginner to commence training the one he finds most congenial and to work for unity and stability in that area. But it is the characteristic of Yoga that all stages are done one after the other and at the same time. For example, right posture, breathing and mental attitude are closely interlinked and interdependent functions.

There are two ways to strengthen *Hara:* one is *Zazen*, or quiet sitting, the other is *Dozen*, or mobile Zen. *Zazen* requires you to devote yourself fully to sitting meditation practice, whilst *Dozen* means to put yourself deliberately into progressively more difficult situations. Because *Dozen* demands your total attention, it develops your ability and raises your consciousness to the highest possible level. This is the process of unification through action and it is the reason why a person who is hovering between life and death has good *Hara*. Both *Zazen* and *Dozen* aim at unifying body and mind and raising consciousness. To *Zazen* and *Dozen* are related *Zengyo* and *kinen*; the ways of discipline and worship, respectively.

Another name for *Zengyo* is *Kensho* and both these terms means experiencing your own maximum potential and being confident that this is possible through your own efforts. As always in Yoga, to attain *Kensho*, it is necessary to discover your own individual discipline and to practice it with the utmost effort. When we realize that we naturally possess deep wisdom and the mysterious ability to physically heal ourselves, it helps us to have the necessary confidence and determination. It took me many years to realize the full implications of this, but in time I saw what the *satori* of the Buddha implies and just how he attained it. By combining the static and the dynamic forms of meditation with the attitudes of self-reliance and worship, we attain the real *Meiso Yoga*.

Whilst I still devoted myself to *Zengyo* solely in order to gain a personal *satori*, I found that the mind remained clouded, dull, and full of guilt, even about simple daily actions. Only when I was able to relinquish self-interest to some extent, through the service of others did *Gudoshin*, "seeking the way through the mind," open up for me. So it was that I entered the way of seeking the truth of life through discipline and worship when the desire for *satori* and salvation wained. I saw that the only way is to take full personal responsibility for grasping the truth and then to apply it to my daily life. When desire for salvation, as something to be acquired, left me, my cancer was healed. It was the most dramatic evidence for the claim that, if the mind is changed, the body will be changed. Although I had carried out physical training almost perfectly, I found that I had not been training the mind. In the course of my experience, I saw that the real way always combines self-reliance, happiness, faith, and deep peace.

(3) The state of Mushin

The condition of consciousness which results from *Zengyo* and *Kinen* is *Mushin*, literally "no-mind." *Mushin* is not vacant mind, however, but the mind of non-attachment which has no prejudice or preference. It is sometimes described as "floating mind" in the sense that consciousness dwells in itself and, from a position of detachment, can observe thoughts and other contents of mind objectively. This is known as apperception and it is the "original" mind which is not limited by fascination with any mental phenomena arising either from external stimulation or from memory. Whereas the worldly mind is totally absorbed by thoughts and so on, the *Mushin* mind remains detached, witnessing their birth and disappearance, yet remaining forever tranquil and detached.

The mind of *Mushin* is also described as being "As bright and clear as a stainless mirror." This analogy refers to the mind's ability to reflect things, yet, like the mirror, to remain without a stain. *Mushin* is also like the surface of a pond which is reflecting the moon. When the moon disappears behind a cloud, the reflection ceases to exist instantly. The worldly mind clings tightly to thoughts and occupies itself with all kinds of emotional reactions long after they would have faded away if they had been left alone. Again, like the surface of a pond into which a stone has been thrown, *Mushin* mind is momentarily disturbed by the passage of thoughts, but instantly returns to silence and peace since it is free and unconditioned.

It is virtually impossible to attain *Mushin* in a single leap, so we make use of the intermediate step of *Isshin*. *Isshin* and *Dharana* closely correspond to each other: the constant practice of concentration ensures that one-pointedness of mind becomes a conditioned reflex. The practice of both *Pratyahara* and *Dharana* trains the mind not to wander and to become focused at will. *Dhyana* frees the mind from attachment and endows it with the ability to be detached from, yet fully open to, all that is. *Dhyana* is actually very easy for a person to attain who is well practiced in *Dharana*. *Dhyana* endows you with the ability to drop one train of thought and instantly devote yourself to another. The faster this change takes place in the mind, the more fluid and adaptable our thinking has become. Such a mind, the mind of *Mushin*, is at the opposite extreme to obsession, for it is a detached state of vivid awareness in which the contents of consciousness are not seized by the mind and, hence, do not dominate. In *Mushin* there may well be thoughts, feelings, and other sense-mediated impressions, but they pass freely through the mind "like birds in the trackless sky."

The symptom of a lack of physical integration is illness, whilst mental problems arise from mental disunity. To attain *satori* is to gain total unity of body and mind and, consequently, to banish physical and mental abnormality. *Mushin* heightens and extends your range of sensation and sharpens your sensibility so that you can see what you could not see before and find more profound truth in life. Because the mind is no longer disturbed by environmental stimulations impinging upon it, the ability to see and evaluate your own mental processes is increased. You will find, to your surprise, that what you had considered "normal" is actually imperfect and abnormal. To change this condition, we must become detached from memory, prejudices and all attachments. We must learn to see with the "naked" mind of *Mushin*. For the worldly mind enmeshed in self-reference, acquisitiveness, knowledge, experience, preconceptions and prejudices are all part of the normal process of judgment. Because of this, we cannot help regarding *Mushin* as something to be gained and so we block our progress by our very efforts to attain.

(4) The condition of Dhyana

Dhyana, or *Mushin*, means that the mind has broken free of the traps which were of its own making and has attained to tranquility and equanimity. In both body and mind, tension and relaxation are now developed to the maximum and, like a gyroscope, the mind is now in a state of dynamic and static balance. Even though a cat is relaxed, it will awaken to the slightest sound and will spring to kill a mouse instantly. So, too, the realized man in the Martial Arts has this cat-like quality of instant readiness. This is also an aspect of *Mushin*, and it is called *Gedatsu*, or release. Contrary to what might be expected, it can be attained without great difficulty by anyone who is well practiced in concentration.

(5) Release and the importance of relaxation

There are two basic styles of meditation, as I have already mentioned. One is the Indian method of isolated practice in relaxation and concentration. The other is the deliberate use of consciously contrived as well as accidental situations of great difficulty in order to develop and unify yourself. The latter is typical of the Chinese and, especially, the Japanese tradition. In this method, considerable tension is induced and much energy is expended by the beginner, so that even sitting for meditation in the Dōjō is full of effort and strain. At this stage, *Dharana* and *Dhyana* are opposite extremes of tension and relaxation, but this difference is progressively reduced and finally eliminated by training. Then, the way we use our energy will have been changed, for it is analogous to a man who is obliged to carry a heavy load. In course of time, he becomes adjusted to the conditions and no longer notices his burden. The point is that maximum tension compels us to attain this dynamic relaxation, so that, even in the midst of seething activity, there is peace. The physiological necessity of alternating periods of tension and relaxation points to the fact that *Dharana* and *Dhyana* follow this natural rhythm. Most people today lack exercise and never develop *Hara* power, which means that they have little energy for relaxing and unifying the body and mind. Because of this, physical strengthening exercises are the vital precondition for effective relaxation and they pay great dividends in return for perseverence. Even though he may be an old man, a person who is used to carrying a heavy load can usually lift more than twice as much as a person who lacks this experience. Through long practice, he has developed his muscles, acquired the best breathing pattern, and developed the best technique. The length of time it takes for these changes to occur means that years are needed to fully master any new practice, including meditation.

Don't Forget to Relax: The *asanas* combine tension and relaxation in natural balance because they are special exercises which were originally developed from meditation. In Japanese, they are called

Zenteki, literally "like Zen." In all things there should be this balance between relaxation and tension and especially so in meditation. To return, briefly, to the analogy of the man who is carrying a heavy load: if he is full of tension, his power will be locked up, but, if he learns to release tension, he can apply all his power to lifting and will find his task easy.

Many people have misconceptions about relaxation, but the following principle is readily recognized to be true. Whatever is done with tension, or is performed hurriedly and with great desire, or anxiety, will seem difficult and unpleasant. This is true even of simple tasks, for whenever we have the wrong attitude, we tire quickly. If such a condition is long continued, or becomes habitual, it leads to abnormality. The best way to overcome this problem is to make a practice of alternating periods of work with periods of rest. This is especially necessary whenever we are required to perform an unfamiliar task, or must give our attention to a particularly important or complex activity. In such cases, we become tense unconsciously and will soon tire. In such situations, we are using muscles and mental functions normally little used, and so we experience apprehension, anxiety, fear, uneasiness and shyness in consequence. The body tries to compensate for this by developing tension, and this absorbs a large proportion of our total energy non-productively. Mind and body quickly become disunified, and confused, and even though we are making maximum exertion, we do not succeed in carrying out the task well.

The best method of relaxing body and mind is not to sleep for long periods, but to alternate short periods of concentrated activity with short periods of rest. The ability to do this depends upon having flexibility of mind, so that it improved remarkably when we practice *Meiso Yoga*. The greatest stamina comes from being able to perform physically demanding activities in a relaxed condition, so that there is a balance of relaxation and tension. Tiredness is a warning signal that immoderate, or unbalanced use is being made of the body, or the mind. Muscles and nerves which are abused suffer from imperfect relaxation and protest by means of the palsy-like condition of tiredness. The whole body should be used, even for small actions which require comparatively little effort. Physical power should flow from the *Hara*, the mind should be relaxed like a smoothly flowing river, and we should rest from time to time.

The right mental attitude towards work is to regard it as play. Both the professional man and the spiritually advanced man work in this way. When work becomes play, all life is relaxation and so there is no need for leisure time or outside diversion. In working and learning, the right way is to prepare the body and mind by means of a "warming-up" period, since this aids you to become centered and to use the whole body. The constant repetition of training is also necessary, of course. In the East, it is said that the students of real *T'ai Chi* and *Shorinji Kempo* were taught nothing about these Martial Arts for at least one year. Then they were required to spend three years learning how to stand and a further three years learning how to walk. This "warming-up" principle was applied to all the arts and skills which are part of the Japanese tradition. Such an approach recognizes the length of time which is needed for real "learning with the body." The student acquired his art not by conceptual analysis but "through the pores of his skin," so to speak. The modern method of education is usually that of teaching techniques. This has two serious disadvantages in that it limits both the development of practical skill and also spiritual progress. The relatively quick acquisition of a technique gives the appearance of changing a person for the better. In fact, however, the person is really unchanged and a ceiling in skill is soon reached, for skill means change. Further, this method reinforces the attitude of "end-gaining," for techniques are useful and profitable acquisitions. As I have already explained, this is a fundamental barrier to spiritual progress.

For these good reasons, no theoretical teaching is given in the Dōjō and no techniques are taught in relation to exercise, healing, or meditation. The student has, therefore, no recourse other than to learn by doing. Tightness of muscle and bad blood condition prevent relaxation. The chief causes of muscle tightness are lack of exercise and poor elimination. Muscle tightness is most apparent on waking in the morning, when the nervous system is slow to work. If the muscles are not used sufficiently, the circulation of hormones in the body is impaired and the muscles become tight in consequence. The nervous system does not work well because of the pressure caused by tight muscles. The more lazy you are, the more you feel disinclined to exercise, whereas, the harder you work, the more flexible your muscles become.

(6) Relaxation of body and mind

The Body: Swinging movements and gentle massage, or patting, makes the body relax. When we ride in a vehicle, such as a car or a train, we easily fall asleep. This fact has traditionally been used to good advantage in the design of the cradle for infants. Quiet, slow movements relax the muscles and nervous system and it is for this reason that a person who is constantly in bed is difficult to heal. There should always be a natural balance between tension and relaxation, for this is the natural rhythm of the body and mind. The more extreme you become in one direction, the more you will need to compensate in the other. Thus, the more timid a person is, the fiercer he will be in a state of fear. So, too, after strong stimulation, or great excitement, the reaction is often a feeling of powerlessness and exhaustion. The best way to relax is to constantly release energy after a spell of tension by breathing deeply and concentrating on the *Hara*. Many people fail to achieve relaxation merely by practicing relaxation techniques because they have not built up sufficient tension to plunge them into the opposite phase of relaxation.

Perfect Yogic breathing also follows a rhythmical pattern of relaxation and tension in alternation. The slight general tension which is natural when you inhale and expand the body should be followed by a short retention of the breath, or *kumbhaka*. On exhaling, the body contracts and there should be a general relaxation. All phases of this Yogic breath should be consciously experienced and controlled until the new pattern becomes habitual. The longer and stronger the exhalation becomes the more relaxed you will be. I have already mentioned that laughter relaxes because it is a naturally prolonged exhalation. It is characteristic of the self-realized person that he can laugh in any situation. In fear, or surprise, we always draw in the breath sharply and become tense. It is not always possible to have a long breath, of course, but by consciously training ourselves to breath abdominally and to relax the upper part of the body, the *Hara* is strengthened and a long breath becomes natural. Chanting, singing, listening to music, and looking at art all help to relax the body and mind and make the breath long.

Mind: It is common experience that we are relaxed when we are doing familiar things and anxious and tense in unfamiliar situations. When you are with people you don't know well, or who seem to have greater ability than yourself, you feel nervous and tense. What has been lost is our normal relaxed breath, but we regain it again as soon as the people concerned are friendly and put us at our ease. We are often tense when waiting for the results of an examination, but it is significant that we relax when the results are known, regardless of the grade we get. It is the unknown which produces tension because our fragile personalities feel more secure in a known and predictable world.

A person who is confident that his illness will be healed, or that his problem can be satisfactorily resolved, has a relaxed and optimistic mind. This is the mind of faith; if faith is grasped and becomes our normal attitude, the mind becomes relaxed. Those who decry faith as being irrational, know neither its real meaning nor its tremendous power. Many religious people acknowledge that faith is rooted in the non-rational level of consciousness, but this is very different from the irrational. Merely because a simple causal explanation of faith is impossible at present, does not mean that faith is unreasonable. Even mathematics and physics today strain the limits of the old rationality and we finally come down to the basic fact that we live together in an organic, interdependent universe. To have faith is to have an unshakable confidence in the ultimately benign nature of the universe and the Life-Force. If this were not true, then there would be no basis for all subsequent rationality.

(7) The worshipful mind

Kinen, literally, "the practice of the praying mind," is the mind which sees, knows and feels God everywhere and is content and happy. This is the practical application of faith and it quickly leads us to *Mushin* and *satori*. Though *Kinen*, we sweep away habit, prejudice and attachments. Following the law of nature, animals live in the state of *Mushin*, but they cannot pray. This is because their minds are not ultimately based upon *satori*. The ability to pray and worship is given only to human beings, whose basic nature is *Bussho*, or natural wisdom. Only human beings can descend into the world of intellect and then regain *Mushin* consciously. This is the privilege of human beings; our lives can be used to contribute some small grain of wisdom to *satori*, for when we regain *Mushin*, we do so wittingly and bring to it our life experience.

When *Bussho*, or natural wisdom, is developed, the mind of worship appears spontaneously and we can accept everything as the love of God and his precious teaching. In this state of mind, the enemy is not an enemy and torture is not torture, for all is teaching. *Kinen*, the practice of the worshipful mind, is to approach the mind of God and to reflect God in your mind. God is love and *Karma*, which makes all things alive; the Life-Force which is far more fundamental than the level of consciousness where we find concepts such as gain and loss, liking and disliking, good and evil. The way of life in which we practice awareness of this level of being is the real religious life.

The worshipful and compassionate mind is born from gratitude and gratitude is expressed as service. On the one hand, *Mushin* means to abolish all limitations of mind through *satori* release, which is the only real freedom. On the other hand, *Kinen* means being able to feel the love of God always and to be able to accept every experience as a valuable training for the benefit of yourself and others. Such a mind does not calculate every situation according to personal advantage and disadvantage. Neither does it take self-reference as the basis of mental and emotional life. This state of mind leads on to the highest tranquility and spiritual ecstasy, which we call *Nirvana*, or Enlightenment.

First Develop the Positive Mind: The mental attitude which generates faith is positive and realistic. To be positive is to emphasize the favorable aspects of every situation. The affirmative mind is quiet and peaceful and takes pleasure in everything. Another basic characteristic of the positive mind is modesty and, in fact, the positive mind is very near to the mind of faith. A self-realized person is one who sees the value of everything that exists and, consequently, respects everyone and everything. He knows that all things appear and disappear in their season due to the necessity of life and so he is not confined to the limited viewpoint of self.

Such a person has gone beyond self because his mind is so positive. Faith does not imply a pessimistic or negative attitude to life. On the contrary, we should always do our utmost and only then, when there is no more to be done, should we leave the rest to God, willingly and completely. This is true tension and relaxation, but in doing your utmost there should be no sense of strain and no arrogance. Even when we are making the greatest efforts, there should be a sense of relaxation and generosity. Only a person who possesses real inner strength can respect everything, apologize for his own failings and continue to work with devotion and appreciation.

(8) Kinen

In Zen discipline, or *Zengyo*, there are two complimentary ways; *Zazen* practice and the life of *Kinen*. *Zazen* aims at attaining stability of mind and body through the practice of sitting meditation. *Kinen* aims at opening yourself to others and to God, so that you may receive his revelations. The character of *Zazen* is given by its objective, the attainment of *Kensho*, or original mind. Similarly, the character of *Kinen* is also derived from its purpose, which is *Kenshin*, or self-sacrifice. Hence we note differences as well as similarities when we compare, say, Japanese religions and Christianity, for although worship and *mantra* are part of *Kinen*, they are also concentrative in effect, like *Dharana*. It is a question of where the basic emphasis is placed in a religion. Whether we choose *Zazen* or *Kinen* depends upon our state of consciousness, for what suits one person may not necessarily suit another. Both ways induce concentration and lead to unity and it may be that most people need both ways at different times in order to attain balance.

(9) Zen, Yoga and Shingon

Both the Zen sect and *Shingon* embody the principles and practices of Yoga; both aim at freedom, Enlightenment and *satori*. Yet it also seems true to say that both lack balance. Zen came from China, where it was strongly influenced by the Taoist way of thought. In some ways, Zen is too religious. Present day Yoga often goes to the opposite extreme and had become overly dependent upon having the truth of its claims confirmed by science. For present purposes, *Shingon* can be classed with Zen, the greatest difference betweeen the two being that, while Zen emphasizes posture, *Shingon* throws all the weight on the unification of the mind through *mantra*.

From the balanced viewpoint of Yoga, Zen imperiously bids us to do what we simply cannot do. Yoga necessarily brings a degree of physical discomfort sometimes, but it regards relaxation as most important and does not compel us to attempt that which is beyond our present capabilities. The disciplines of meditation and worship, for example, are not introduced until the student has gained confidence and competence. Even though the beginner may be taught to adopt the posture of *Zazen*, he has no ability to stand detached from the thought-stream and so *Zazen* is really of little use to him. Yoga begins at ground level, carefully preparing the body and mind before introducing meditation. The beginner may certainly practice sitting but is not expected to embark upon serious meditation for some time. Present day Zen has no policy of healing and strengthening the physical body before embarking upon mind training. Yoga is influenced by the theory of rebirth and *Karma*; the character of people in Yoga is marked by patience and an air of leisure. Zen accurately reflects the Japanese character, which is very different. The Japanese are intensely active and prefer to die gallantly rather than live in ignominy. In some ways, the thinking of *Soto* Zen is nearer to Yoga than that of *Rinzai* Zen because it teaches that *satori* should be ap-

The Seventh Stage / 117

proached patiently and gradually and that the wisdom of Zen should be incorporated into our daily life. But even *Soto* lacks the logical and progressive sequence of stages which characterizes Yoga.

(10) About Yoga and Shingon Yuga

The word *Yuga*, used in *Shingon* esoteric Buddhism is simply a transliteration of the word *Yoga*. One who trains in Yoga is called a *yugasha* in Japanese, but *Shingon* makes use of the term *Shingon-gyoja*. The original *Shingon* Dōjō was established on Mount Koya, in western Japan, about one thousand years ago by the monk, Kūkai. *Shingon* practice is based upon the *Kongoho Rokaku Issai Yuga Yugikyo*, an esoteric sutra. The *Shingon* Dōjō is a vital, living link with the Yoga of ancient times, for Kūkai learnt his *Shingon* teaching from China, whence it had been brought from Tibet. Tibetan esoteric Buddhism had four schools, the *Kuriya*, the *Karma*, the *Yoga*, and the *Anitara Yoga*. Although we know relatively little about their practices, we can infer that the Yoga of the period was centered on disciplines for guarding the senses and developing concentration. In India, the *Katha Upanisad* described Yoga as seeking the union of *Atman* and *Brahman*, subject and object. Indeed, there is a basic similarity between some phases of Indian Yoga and *Shingon*, despite the great differences of time and place. The great power behind the universe of appearances, called *Brahman* in India, becomes *Dainichi Nyorai* in *Shingon*. No matter what name is used, it is the real essence of all things, the Life-Force, or God, of Yoga. Yoga aims to release consciousness from the limitations of individual existence and to re-unite it with the greater principle. *Shingon* esoteric Buddhism thus continues ancient and original Yoga in a Buddhistic form. If we exclude the crudely physical schools of *Hatha Yoga*, we find in *Shingon* all the main factors of Yoga, such as meditation, *mantra*, supra-mental experience, philosophy and logic. Yoga continues to influence many Buddhist sects and even the *mantra* of the Nichiren sect is Yogic in origin. Nichiren himself split off from *Tendai* esoteric Buddhism, which had much in common with *Shingon*. Nichiren's *mantra*, *Namu Myoho Renge Kyo*, means that individual and social harmony can arise only from the insight that all men are brothers. It is a Yogic sentiment expressed through a Yogic practice. I intend to explain more fully about *Shingon* in the second volume of *Meiso Yoga*.

(11) The Way of Hannya

Meditation brings about the union of intellect with the body, senses, and emotions. When this union is attained, real wisdom can be grasped. To explain this, it is necessary to consider man's relationship to his environment. Scientists assure us that, long, long ago, life existed only in the form of single living cells like the ameba. At that level, life is fully dependent upon instinct, so that the ameba's life is a function of nature, or the universe. The ameba is not taught, yet it knows what is suitable for it in terms of food, environment and so on. The same natural wisdom which the ameba possesses is present also in human beings.

Human beings also inherit traits and tendencies from their ancestors which is like a sort of racial memory incorporated in their cells. They reproduce skills, such as walking, which emerge in them as children when they reach a certain stage of development. In addition to these factors, there is *Reikan*—"soul-feeling," intuition, or inspiration. Instincts, traits, and intuition amount to the original mind which is given at birth. It generates the desire for life which brings about birth and the wisdom which emerges from the unconscious levels of mind.

There was a time when life on this planet existed only in the oceans. The memory of that experience is also carried in our cells and the human embryo still begins life in water. All our innate abilities derive from the experience of the past and human beings seem to go through an individual development which mirrors that of the race. Now, this deep wisdom of the original mind does not depend upon ratiocination or teachings, but arises spontaneously from the beginning. This is seen clearly when we recognize that, even though we understand in detail how human beings are born, we are unable to give birth to new life merely by virtue of this knowledge.

Thus we already possess this deep wisdom of nature for which knowledge is no substitute. If you really grasp this point you can scarcely avoid a feeling of gratitude to nature, the universe and to our ancestors. Most people accept the fact of their own existence in a purely matter of fact manner, but our present life is really something of a miracle, not to appreciate this is dull and unimaginative. The realization that your life is the product of the effort and cooperation of your ancestors and of the entire universe generates a deep sense of gratitude and worship. In the philosophy of totality, which characterizes Yoga and Buddhism, it is recognized that we did not make ourselves and even the intellect is far from autonomous and independent. In all that we do, say, and think, we have a debt of gratitude to others and a very real and deep responsibility.

(12) Helping Hannya and Reikan to develop

Part of the purpose of *Meiso Yoga* is to make us more sensitive to the voice of the original mind which we call wisdom, or intuition. Through *Meiso Yoga* you will see the wisdom of all things and you will see how the universe pours and melts into the rational mind. When we learn to cooperate with the truth of our real situation, we experience *Mushin* and *satori*. Then it is that *Atman* and *Brahman*, true self and God, become one. The basic character of human beings is that of a thinking animal. To increase our humanity it is not sufficient, therefore, only to develop thought. If we are one-sided and ignore the original mind of natural wisdom, our humanity can never fully emerge. Through *Hannya*, the universal mind pervades the intellect and dissolves the prejudice and attachment of the worldly mind. The entire purpose of the universe is to refine consciousness through human experience and to make human beings divine. The difficulty of providing a precise definition of *Hannya* springs from the fact that words are the product of the rational mind. *Hannya* is deeper, wider, and more profound than rationality and so the only way to grasp it is with the whole body-mind organism. The great sutra of *Mahayama* Buddhism, the *Maka Hannya Haramita Shingyo*, teaches us the deep truth of *Hannya* through its powerful spiritual vibrations. Although it is the shortest of all Buddhist sutras, the real teaching of the Buddha is found here in its essence.

5. Satori: The Eighth and Highest Stage

When individual consciousness is unconditioned and empty of contents, it becomes one with all consciousness. Instead of being the necessarily limited consciousness of this or that individual, it becomes itself. It is no longer consciousness of this or that object, but has become the universal principle of consciousness and all is seen from a very different point of view. Now, everything is self and, hence, everything is valuable. The whole world glows with a strange new light. This is the condition of *satori*: that in this state "I myself" pours and melts into all objects and no longer exists as a limited, separate principle. *Satori* proves that the difference between self and other can become unnecessary when mind regains its original state. Only in *satori* can we know and express true love.

Love is the law of nature and the mind of the universe, or God. The true expression of love is to make oneself and others more and more alive and to share prosperity together. When we can live this truth, the true Enlightenment is given. *Satori* is attained by losing self in the service of others and then going on to that sanctification of mind called Enlightenment, which is the highest and most divine condition. The *Meiso Yoga*, practiced by the Buddha and the Christ, is the only Path to this state. In Enlightenment, man becomes God and God becomes man. Such a divine being looks benignly upon the world, seeing the true value of all beings shining forth as a strange, supernatural light. He can enter into the mind of any being, understanding and sympathizing with any point of view.

(1) Bhakti and Karma Yoga

As well as *Raja Yoga*, the disciplines of *Bhakti* and *Karma Yoga* are also ways to Enlightenment. The theater of *Karma Yoga* is our daily life and work; in Zen it is called *samugyo*, or "work training."

Karma Yoga means living a life in which your self-interest and personal pleasure is not different to that of others. Through this commonality of interest we can make others, little by little, more alive which is a kind of mutual worship. In Yoga, it becomes impossible to regard either life or work as being exclusively your own, or to think of your job as a mere job.

Karma Yoga teaches us that work should be our training ground for receiving and expressing love and for attaining *satori*. Your job should be the medium through which you can express your gratitude to God and to other people for what they have done for you. It should never be "mere work." Life itself is our most precious possession and is indeed worthy of our worship as we strive to attain the ideal life and society. *Karma Yoga* can be a training in concentration and detachment as well as service. As you work, phenomena appear and disappear. We can learn detachment by concentrating on the efficient performance of our duties, but we must not forget common human warmth and kindness in the process. When you approach your work with this faith, you can offer your mind and body completely in the service of others. The *satori* of work is attained when we become the perfect expression of the values and abilities which our job demands; in other words, when "I" and "job" become one. *Satori* should not be thought of as some kind of useless ecstasy or rapture, or even as a hypnotic trance; it is quite different. When a person is in *satori*, his body and mind are very flexible and tranquil, but his awareness of his surroundings is actually far keener than usual. Consequently, a person in *satori* can adapt, easily and rapidly, to changing circumstances, for there is nothing that he does not enjoy from the bottom of his heart. Ecstasy is quite different, for it is a condition in which you cannot react to any stimuli from the environment because consciousness is totally indulged in one thing. Ecstasy is thus the supreme selfishness. In *satori*, you can do everything, freely and voluntarily, which is very different from the state of ecstasy. Now, although I have tried my best to describe *satori*, I must finally say that it is beyond description. *Satori* is the synthesis, or culmination, of all our previous training. Even though we might have an excellent intellectual grasp of *satori*, we still cannot know it except by experiencing it ourselves. That experience can be ours only when we have regained a natural body and a purified mind.

(2) About Karma Yoga

I have already explained that, in *Karma Yoga, satori* means that condition in which you are able to make yourself and others more fully alive through your work. To do this we must work with the detachment of *Mushin*. One of the ways that we employ in Okidō to bring people to *satori* is the training through work. Human beings can work at different levels of consciousness, however, and this affects their mental and physical condition. True work is very different, for example, from the lowest level, which I call *Rodo*. *Rodo* corresponds to the level of a paid laborer and amounts to no more than wage-slavery. This relationship to work degrades human beings to the level of animals, for it is only an exchange of your physical and mental strength for the essentials of life. The working person is thus encouraged by the conditions of his employment to seek to reduce working hours to the minimum and increase his financial reward to the maximum.

The entire concept of wage-labor seems to me to be an expression of the Puritan mentality which influenced the industrial revolutions of both England and America. Like Puritanism itself, the concept of wage-labor lacks balance. Human relationships are subordinated to the employment contract and natural pleasure in work is destroyed by the extreme application of the principle of the division of labor. Present day labor movements only compound this inhuman system because they operate only within the logic of the employment situation. The quality of life of employees cannot be improved merely by higher wages and shorter hours, for such adjustments only intensify the conflict inherent in wage-labor. The only worthwhile answer is to change the entire basis of employment and this can be done through *Karma Yoga*. Puritanism began as a genuinely religious movement, but it lost its soul to capitalism. It is yet another example of the fact that true spirituality cannot survive the embrace of power and wealth. The result of this loss of spirituality in the West is a society which has created anti-human conditions for itself. Human dignity is destroyed by the employment relationship and human activity is devalued as a result of the division of labor.

One of the most tragic results of this situation is that few people today have any real purpose in life beyond the acquisition of wealth and possessions. Life becomes more and more unnatural because the end-product of so much of our labor is either incredibly trivial, or non-existent. It is only natural, therefore, that people have little interest in their work and little sense of social responsibility for what they produce. Within the present debased concept of labor it is actually logical to be concerned only with the material returns for sacrificing a significant portion of your life to a restricting and boring situation. Wage labor does not even represent a true materialism in which people have leisure to enjoy materials and material pleasures. It is diametrically opposed to *satori*, for it produces only the disunity of the self and the disunity of society. It alienates human beings from nature. Rather than being rewarded by a creative materialism, people are de-energized and emasculated in order to prevent them from rebelling against the system. The many temptations which society offers and to which it gives its implicit approval are invitations to compensate yourself for the evils of the employment system by indulging the instinctive desires. This strengthens our dependence upon the present social order and distorts our true human nature.

About Kido—the Way of Pleasure in Work: The foregoing may paint too dark a picture, for even nowadays there are many people who enjoy their work. They are people who voluntarily dedicate themselves to their job. Such a condition is similar to *Kido* but is still not the real thing. It is actually a form of selfishness, for such people will often sacrifice anyone and anything for personal success in their jobs. For example: those industrialists who ignore the social cost of production processes which pollute the environment are in this category. Real *Kido* is attained when you derive pleasure from the work itself, from the pleasure of others in the work, and from the pleasure of the consumers in your products. *Kido* is a step upwards in the process of upgrading work to the level required by *Karma Yoga.*

About Shado—the Way of Gratitude in Work: After *Kido* comes *Shado*. In former times, Japanese people naturally felt that they wanted to express their gratitude to others through their work. The Japanese word for work is *hataraku*: *hata* means "surroundings" including other people, and *raku* means "comfortable." Thus *hataraku* means "to make others comfortable" and it implies a very different basis for work than wage-labor. The concept of work at one time included these ideas of service and consideration for others as the basic motivation; personal gain was secondary. This way of thinking is the religious attitude to work.

About Etsudo—the Way of Merging with Work: Following *Shado* comes *Etsudo* in which the mind melts into the mind of God and work becomes the most profound delight. This is the most noble state of work in which you and the work become one. Through your work "I" becomes other and thus the whole of society. The reward for your labors is the gratitude and admiration of other. There is no personal pride involved, however, because you are aware that many hidden factors have cooperated to make this condition possible. It is *Karma Yoga* in action, the ideal Yogic way of life. *Etsudo* is *satori* in action.

When asked about prayer, I always advise people to pray through their work and for their work, but few understand the way of prayer. Prayer does not mean asking for what you want, but asking for what others need. It means beseeching God to use you and your work to help other people. The mind of prayer arises from *Mushin*, for true prayer is empty of thoughts of self. It is the mind which is devoid of concepts and is therefore unconditioned. The mind of prayer does not regard service as charity, makes no calculations about profit and loss and keeps no record of services rendered. It is non-judgmental, yet works with gratitude, real enjoyment, and total commitment.

(3) Hoetsu: Enlightenment

Enlightenment is Sacred pleasure and pure religious ecstasy. It is a stage of Yoga even further advanced than *satori*. Although it is not included in the classical formulations of the eight stages of Yoga, I believe that it is the highest attainment of the Yogin. After *satori* has been experienced, divine pleasure gushes forth through body and mind and the entire world is transformed into a pure paradise. When the Buddha attained Enlightenment, he cried out spontaneously that all is goodness and pleasure.

No-one should ever feel that *satori* is too high for them to attain. We should all model ourselves on the example of the Buddha and the Christ, for that is what they wanted. If we use every incident in our daily life as a training in awareness and pray constantly that our work will help others along the way we shall easily succeed. This way of life arouses the original mind of nature and leads us directly to *Mushin* and *satori*. Out of this awareness, a genuine sense of penitence is born and those habits of ours which injure living beings, however indirectly, will fall away. We can gradually perfect ourselves if we take the great religious teachers as our example and practice Yoga. Let us take this way together.

The spiritual life of Yoga is *Mikkyo*, or esoteric religion. *Mikkyo* means to grasp the truth by your own efforts and as a result of your own experience. However, this can easily be misunderstood. It does not mean that everyone can do as they like, for that would be a kind of anarchy. Although Yoga makes full allowance for individuality, we must follow the outlines of a specific path unconditionally and without reluctance, until we attain *satori*. The lives of the holy teachers of mankind are our best guide.

Chapter 4 Personal Experiences

I. Meiso Yoga in the Dōjō

Those who have not experienced Dōjō life cannot know how meditation fits into the pattern of daily life nor how it relates to other training. We must always remember that the final goal of Yoga training is meditation; indeed that is why Yoga is Yoga. *Asana, Pranayama,* and so on, are part of a process leading to meditation and, if we forget this and devote ourselves to meditation alone, our Yoga practice will be unbalanced. Unless you have balance in your daily life as well as during the actual practice of Yoga, significant effects cannot be expected. As a specific example of the Yogic lifestyle, I am here decribing the Dōjō day in which every event contributes to the purpose of mastering Yoga. If you can understand the principles behind this program it will help you to integrate meditation into your daily life. If this section is approached in this spirit, it will form a good manual for your Yoga study before you go to an Okidō Dōjō.

All the details and rules of the Dōjō training have been voluntarily worked out by the trainees. The underlying purpose is to encourage the student to overcome reluctance and to take personel responsibility for his own development. It leads to self-mastery through giving you the opportunity to impose your own autonomous discipline. Although the Dōjō program is strictly followed, the students have much free time in order that they can adapt themselves to the new way of life. The essential principles embodied in the Dōjō life are the alternation of concentration and release, warmth and cold, tension and relaxation, intake and elimination. By obeying the natural laws of exchanging materials with the universe, of prayer, service, laughter and enjoyment, the mind and body are prepared for a higher level of performance. The pattern of Dōjō life can be adapted to accord with your job and other commitments in daily life. As you read on, try to appreciate the real meaning and rhythm of the schedule.

Seeking the truth through Yoga must extend into all aspects of your life and your job, especially, must be seen as Yoga because it takes up so much of your time. That is the true *satori* training of Zen which is taught in Okidō. According to this teaching, recreation is also Yoga training and so are sleeping and eating. This is the way to really make the best of yourself and get the most out of life. If you try to make your whole life Yoga training, the effect on you will be several times greater than otherwise. The essence of Yoga training is to have a deep purpose and not to be contented with mere physical training. I hope that all my readers will take this to heart and begin a total dedication of themselves to seeking the truth.

Awaking: There are occasions when we, in the Dōjō, get up very early, but usually we rise at five or five-thirty in the morning. Most people then follow cleansing and stimulating techniques, such as a cold water wash and rubbing their bodies with a dry towel. Whenever a training activity is begun or ended in the Dōjō, we make it a rule to do *Gassho* and repeat the appropriate vow. Since all activities are a training for us, vows are repeated a lot. Now, although this may appear to be childish, this practice has certain valuable effects. Frequent chanting improves the breathing, whilst the prayer-like *Gassho* posture spreads the chest, stretches the spine and lowers the center of gravity of the body to the *Hara*. There is a psychological advantage, too, for to say the vow to yourself is to clarify the principles which guide your daily life and to reaffirm your ultimate purpose. Such mental activity liberates the spirit from the mundane affairs of life and makes it far easier to raise the level of consciousness. The raising of consciousness is what you should aim at in all phases of your life.

Awakening Vow

"We give thanks for our awakening. Awakening means that we have received the blessing of sufficient physical strength to live. We vow that this day we will bring all our strength to everything we do in order to live."

Through Yoga, we aim to develop our full potential as persons and to express our ability in accordance with natural law and the rhythm of the universe. By devoting yourself totally to whatever you are doing at the moment, you are giving active proof of your faith in God. In consequence, God will give the result, for it is simply the life of doing your best and utilizing your total ability. Yoga teaches us that awakening proves that we still have life and consciousness. It is our total concern to do everything possible to ensure that consciousness is awake, lucid and clear.

Sometimes, you may suddenly become objectively aware that you have life and think to yourself "Oh! here I am, alive." That is a good experience which arises when all the small functions of the body are working with full individual efficiency and when the total system is in a state of harmony and balance. It is especially important that a person who is seriously ill should realize that, insofar as he is alive, he has also been given the power to heal himself. The Japanese word *Arigato* literally means "there is much difficulty." Whatever is given to us by others should not be taken for granted, for the combined efforts of many people as well as the beneficent forces of nature have all contributed to its presence now before you. Life manifests through miraculously-made complex organic systems and we should, in all humility, be grateful that life has been given to us.

The awakening vow seeks to express awareness of the cooperation of countless factors to provide us with materials and opportunity. If religious language seems too humble, we should reflect that it helps us to realize our true relationship with the universe. By regular repetition of the sacred words of religion we can establish gratitude and thankfulness as a permanent attitude of mind. This will serve as a warning signal which will prevent us from working against the order of the universe. If we practice serene detachment and recognize that thoughts, emotions and so on, only arise and fall in the mind, then we can adapt ourselves effortlessly to any situation.

It may well be that the reader will readily agree with what I have said and even make notes of the important points. At some future time, you may actually recall these ideas although you temporarily forgot them in between. Human beings are weak and forgetful and so the daily repetition of the pledges with *Gassho* performs an invaluable function.

Cleaning and Dokkyo: About six o'clock in the morning, all the students in the Dōjō commence a cleaning routine. This itself is a training because it is a golden opportunity to practice natural body movement. Cleaning the rooms is an extension of the purifying activities we engage in for some time after awakening. It is purification of the environment.

Cleaning Vow

"We will now take part in the training of cleaning. We vow to cleanse the body, the mind and the environment. The purified mind does not desire. It is the mind to serve others and to fully appreciate life."

Here I will explain how to do *Gassho* correctly whilst chanting the vow. *Gassho* is a *mudra* which combines the joining of the hands and of the legs. It is one of the *mudras* used in esoteric *Shingon*. There are several hundred *mudras* and the posture and breathing is different in each. There are many variations of *Gassho* and here I describe only the basic form.

First sit in *Seiza* or any crossed-leg position, then bring the hands tightly together so that there is contact from the finger tips to the heel of the hands. Release all tension from the shoulders, make the forearms horizontal and hold the tips of the index fingers level with the eyes. Stretch the neck and spine upwards, press the hands together and do rhythmical *Hara* breathing whilst consciously putting power in the abdomen. Concentrate attention on the tips of the index fingers and hold a mental image of the ideal state you wish to attain. When repeating the pledge, try to hold the meaning of the words in mind.

After cleaning, all the students gather to practice *Dokkyo*. This is the Japanese word for chanting and the sutra we chant is the *Hannya Shinkyo*. We try to concentrate our attention totally on the words of the sutra and not to indulge in random thoughts. From the point of view of breathing, it is important to chant for as long as possible on each breath so as to exhale fully. In the Dōjō there are from three to seven periods of chanting every day. The usual clothing worn is a loose fitting training suit.

Marathon and Cold Bath: After *Dokkyo* everyone goes jogging along the country lanes. Each person must decide his own limits, however, and whilst some run ten kilometers others begin to walk after only one hundred meters. They run fast or slow according to individual ability and condition. Marathon is a training as well as physical exercise and the main point of it is to change the breathing. Everyone must discover his own best stride, posture and movement. The body should be held erect, the chest expanded and the shoulders lowered. The movement should flow from the *Hara* center down through the hips and legs. There is a similarity between the right posture for running and that of *Zazen*. The leg and arm movements are coordinated and there is controlled and rhythmical breathing. Each person discovers what is the most suitable way of breathing for himself. In marathon there is exercise and movement as well as *asana*. Yoga students treat it as a form of Zen exercise, concentrating their attention on the movements and their state of mind.

Marathon strengthens the legs and the waist if they have become weak. Strength in these places relates directly to *Hara* power and good blood circulation. It also helps to develop the vital coordination between the legs and the upper body. Sometimes people experience a lack of coordination when they want to hurry and the legs refuse to move quickly enough. In extreme cases they experience the body as a group of almost unrelated parts rather than as a total organism. Marathon helps to overcome these problems for it develops all the body and increases stamina. As I have said, we need a rhythm of alternating warmth and cold as well as tension and relaxation. After the body has become hot through running it is good to take a cold bath. The Dōjō students sometimes go under a nearby waterfall, but whether we bathe indoors or outdoors we should never jump into the water as the shock can be dangerous to the heart.

First splash the hands and feet and enter into the water slowly. All our activities in the Dōjō are intended to purify both body and mind. We vow to eliminate both mental and physical poisons. After marathon, we attend to necessary work for the Dōjō. Each person must try to be constantly aware in everything he does and is helped in this by the practice of writing a daily report. This practice promotes self-reflection and, in consequence, the desire to change various aspects of character.

Satori Training: After purifying exercises, we engage in service. That is, we do jobs of many kinds about the Dōjō. Sometimes we do construction work, or agricultural work in the fields. One person might be carrying earth whilst another will be writing articles on Yoga for the Dōjō magazine. The original Yoga Dōjō at Mishima was built entirely by the trainees themselves. This kind of work is real *satori* training when it is used as an opportunity to forget self-interest. If we can become one with the work we can bring it to life with a tremendous surge of creativity. In that state we have no desire for reward because the satisfaction of the job itself is reward enough. It is then that the real pleasure of work becomes known.

The Morning Vow and Kyokaho: About 11.00 A.M. everyone assembles for *Asa No Aisatsu*, or morning greeting. Sometimes a short talk is given on a current topic, whilst on other occasions students take turns in expressing their views on some issue of general community interest. Often too, the previous day's reports provide a specific personal problem which can be used as the occasion for teaching basic principles. Through this process, each person is helped to come to his own self-understanding in Okidō.

After the morning greeting, the students do either *Kyokaho* or *Shuseiho*, according to individual need. *Kyokaho* are strengthening exercises whilst *Shuseiho* are special corrective exercises. The purpose of *Kyokaho* is not simply physical exercise but, more importantly, to help to create a positive and unified mind. It is also a form of diagnostic technique which reveals the true condition of each person. *Kyokaho* includes such activities as moving hand over hand along a roof beam, climbing ropes, or performing various techniques adapted from the martial arts. Although the training is hard, I am proud of the fact that no-one is ever seriously injured. The vital thing in *Kyokaho* is to learn to take an intense interest in what is actually happening and to perform all the activities positively and with laughter. From the point of view of the teacher, *Kyokaho* allows the observation of every student individually. My diagnosis of their real condition is based upon at least four phases of human behavior.

$$\text{Posture} \begin{cases} \text{Conscious} \begin{cases} \text{mobile} \\ \text{static} \end{cases} \\ \text{Unconscious} \begin{cases} \text{mobile} \\ \text{static} \end{cases} \end{cases}$$

During the fast moving activity of *Kyokaho*, I am able to see the students reacting in a variety of ways to difficult and unfamiliar situations. The students themselves quickly become aware of their weak points and are thereby enabled to take positive corrective action.

The Vow of Kyokaho

"I have seen that body and mind are strengthened by correct training and I realize that only training will allow me to express my full ability as a person. To become an agent of pure love who can give selfless service and real cooperation to others, I shall do *Kyokaho* with my whole body and mind. I vow to be of positive mind, to reject complaint and to endure cheerfully. There shall be no resentment or reluctance in me."

Those who do not do *Kyokaho* engage in *Shuseiho*. There are different types of corrective exercises according to whether the fault to be corrected is long-standing or recent. *Shuseiho* is a science in its own right and the reader can learn more about it from my book *Healing Yourself Through Okidō Yoga*.

The Vow of Shuseiho

"The art of life is the art of maintaining balance. Distorted minds and bodies are the result of the wrong way of life which destroys that balance. I vow to devote myself fully to *Shuseiho* to correct distortions and so to regain balance and harmony."

Perhaps seven hours have now passed since awakening and so it is time to take a rest. The first substantial meal is taken about 12.30 P.M., for breakfast consists of only a bowl of *miso* soup. Many people find difficulty in adhering to this dietary regime at first, but soon become used to living on only two meals a day. If you eat only the food which is suitable for you as an individual, a large quantity is unnecessary.

The Vow of Nutrition

"The meaning of nutrition is to absorb the good and reject the unnecessary. It is within the power of the body, through its innate wisdom, to distinguish the necessary from the superfluous."

After lunch, we often do laughing exercises for five or ten minutes. The effects of this were explained earlier. Then we take a well-earned rest for about two hours. After meals, relaxation is necessary and I have often noticed that primitive people know intuitively that it is right to sleep after meals. I personally find that a short sleep of about twenty minutes is enough. After resting, many people like to go out into the countryside to receive the beauty of nature. This, too, can be a valuable practice in choiceless acceptance, for to receive nature with a pure mind is to receive spiritual food. Others prefer to play sports, do personal jobs, or simply go out for a walk.

Individual Training and Lectures: When the students return about 4.00 P.M. they select their activities according to their preference and physical condition. Options such as massage, acupuncture, martial arts, flower arranging, tea-ceremony, traditional dancing, Japanese sung poetry, sauna bath, or natural hot-spring bath are sometimes available. All these activities should be seen as training for the mind and the breath. They should be used as invaluable opportunities to make the greatest possible use of materials and objects. About 5.30 P.M. lectures begin and are usually concerned with the physiological aspects of Yoga.

Supper and Evening Relaxation: About 6.30 P.M. the second meal of the day is served. It consists of a bowl of buckwheat noodles and soy soup. It is the last meal of the day and it is a surprising fact that many students find that it is not necessary. After supper, the students can chose between hot, cold, herbal, steam or sauna baths according to their preference and needs. About 8.00 P.M. we have singing and there is always much laughter. These occasions are comparable to the communal festivals of primitive tribal society. In the daytime there is tension, but at night-time there is relaxation and a friendly atmosphere. Even this is a training, however, for it gives everyone the opportunity to become open and sociable. At such times we owe it to others to be good companions even if we feel like being silent and reticent. After the singing there is an evening meeting in which opinions are frankly expressed and problems discussed. The solutions to personal problems are often found at these meetings, for the whole purpose of them is to help people in their search for self-understanding.

Meditation Exercise at Night: About 9.00 P.M. we have meditation exercise for about thirty or forty minutes. The first half of this period is devoted to concentration exercises and the second half to the practice of *Mu*-mind. After meditation, there is usually a lecture which lasts until about 10.00 P.M. The daily program is now at an end but each student must write a report on his day's activities before going to bed. In this way, activity and reflection, body and mind are trained to become one. This is the way of Yoga.

The Vow of Meditation

"The best human condition is that which is natural. What is natural is harmonious. When we have harmony we are stable and tranquil. Human beings easily fall into the unbalanced state of partial, small-minded views and unwise attachments, however. It is vital to maintain balance by consciously counteracting this tendency. In meditation we train both mind and body in serene detachment. I vow that in this meditation I will reach towards the purity of emptiness."

Before the students retire for the night, one more vow is made. It is the *Vow of Rest*.

The Vow of Rest

"I am grateful for all the good things I have received today, especially the privilege of life itself. I am conscious of my deep indebtedness to the living universe for the opportunities and knowledge I have been given. Tomorrow will be another precious opportunity and I vow to do even better. Now I shall permit myself to rest in the clear awareness of gratitude and the quiet determination to improve in every way."

The daily schedule I have described is constantly changed so that nothing can become habitual. The principles upon which it is based can be used to transform your daily life into an effective Yoga training. Perhaps the first principle is to follow all physical activities as a form of mind-training through detachment, lack of concern for personal profit, and the will to be of service.

2. The Sacred in Gaol—The Teaching of Hoseini-shi

The Difficulties of Entering into Spiritual Training: I want to explain here how I came to enter into training and what brought me to the life of seeking the truth. Firstly I had unusual experience right from infancy, for virtually the first words I learnt were the words of the *Nembutsu* and my father taught me *Zazen* when I was only five years old. My schoolmaster at Junior High School used to let us come to school an hour before lessons started so that we could do *Zazen* every day. Yet despite this training in practicing without thinking or doubting, I used to ask my parents and teacher "What is the purpose of sitting?" and "What will happen if I chant the *Nembutsu?*" My teacher replied "Anyway sit. *Zazen* refreshes you in body and mind. Believe in this and just follow." I had the feeling that I was better when I did *Zazen* than when I did not. Still I could not really understand the meaning of prayer and Zen training, but my doubts were what brought me to the serious practice of chanting and meditation later in my life.

One of the great turning points of my life was in 1939 when the Second World War was about to break out. I was selected as a special agent of Section 2 of the General Staff Office and later sent to Mongolia and the Middle East. My appointed task was to enter South Asia and the southern part of China and to cooperate with the independence movement of Mohammedans in those areas. The first step was to go to Tibet and so I was given a special training in a Buddhist monastery in Mongolia for about eight months. So that my cover would be convincing, I trained myself to be a real Lama. This might seem to have been a strange religious experience, but my chief motive was always to serve my country as a spy. It was not really a religious experience for me. Conditions in that monastery would have appalled most civilized people, for neither clothing nor cooking utensils were ever washed and most of the monks had suffered from syphilis since birth.

In time I became accustomed to the life and even memorized the chanting, although I didn't know the meaning of the words. In later years I realized what a valuable experience it had been and felt that it had probably worked out for the best. Because I was acting a part, I devoted myself to study with more effort than the Lamas themselves! It was the memory of the teachers of my childhood and what they had taught me about Buddhism that enabled me to enter into my role and endure the difficulties of life. When I was returning from Tibet, the route lay across a desert and we rode on camels for about fifty days. At one point we were attacked by fierce tribesmen and my party was dispersed. I took refuge in a mosque, which was my first contact with Islam. It was a useful experience, for when I later returned to Japan, I received the special assignment to work with the Mohammedan independence movements. My route lay through India where I visited a Yoga ashram and had contact with Yogins. At that time I had no idea that I would become a Yogin in the future. Whilst in India, I also chanced to meet Mahatma Gandhi for the first time. The reason why I went to India was to enter Iran, for the two countries were on friendly terms, and from Iran to infiltrate into Central Asia and Southern China. At that time the governments of Turkey and Iran had a common policy of oppressing Islam and they prohibited foreigners from making contact with religious people. Unfortunately my attempts to make secret contact with the head of Islam in Iran were detected and subsequently I was followed by government agents wherever I went. I escaped to Iraq for a time but later entered Iran once again. I found that my contacts had all left by that time and I was unable to find a place of security. Some time later, I was arrested and put in gaol in the suburbs of Meshed in the north-east of Iran, near to Russia and South Asia. In that gaol I was compelled to wear a leg chain about two meters long at the end of which was an iron ball about sixty centimeters in diameter.

My Friend in Gaol: After being in gaol for about twenty days a new prisoner joined me. He was a very quiet, refined old gentleman in Persian dress and when he entered my cell I had a strange feeling that the thick walls had melted away. He seemed to be actually enjoying his predicament, for his face was always serene and peaceful. I noticed that he did not have a leg chain and wondered if he had occupied some important position. One day I asked him in my

The Sacred in Gaol—The Teaching of Hoseini-shi / 139

limited Persian—
"Why havn't they given you a leg chain?"
He replied in fluent English, which I could understand—
"Because my punishment is already fixed and because I am a man of religion."
I asked him if his punishment was long-term imprisonment? He replied—
"My punishment is death."
Then he asked me—
"How about you? I hear you were a smuggler and that you were arrested by the Chinese."
I replied—
"No, I am a Japanese and I've never been a smuggler."
He said that it was quite rare to meet a Japanese in that part of the world. I asked him—
"Why are they going to execute you? Did you kill someone?"
"No," he said, "I was against the policy of the Emperor, so the government found me guilty of inciting rebellion."
He said this with a very evident feeling of pleasure, as if he had been given a prize. I felt that he was living in a very different world and wondered if he was mad. I said to him—
"Your English is very good, where did you learn it?"
He replied that he had studied in India, France, Germany and England since he was fifteen years old.
At no time did my friend offer me any information unless I asked him a question and, although he was sitting next to me, I felt that he was not really there. Sometimes he chanted a prayer several times and I began to wonder if it was all a pose to hide his fear of death. He might be using *mantra* and meditation merely to prevent himself thinking about the terrible position he was in.
But his manner continued to be very warm and peaceful, yet solemn, and I gradually became ashamed to have entertained such doubts. His eyes were bright and happy looking and never showed timidity or agony. I could see nothing at all in his actions which indicated anxiety; he did not sigh or yawn, nor did he rub his hands together nervously. He just continued to sit in a tranquil way, re-

minding me constantly of the Buddha. After I had sat besides him for a long time I had a strong impression that he was surrounded by light. I already had a deep respect for him and did not find it difficult to believe that what I saw was the nimbus which is said to have appeared about the head of the Buddha and the Christ.

Later, I asked him—

"You are going to be executed, yet you seem to be utterly at peace. Have you resolved the problem of death? If I can give up everything will I be like you?"

He replied—"Give up? What must you give up? You told me before that your mind is ready to accept anything that might happen. If you force yourself to give up what you believe in, or to make some unnecessary decision, your mind will be false and easily corrupted."

The old man had seen that my resolution was false because it was based only upon a rational decision. I felt that I too might be executed and, feeling anxious, I asked him—

"What kind of mind should I have?"

He replied like a Zen Master—

"Usual mind. I think it is only natural that we have thoughts according to the situation and our surroundings. You ask me how I can be happy in this gaol? It is natural for me to feel fear, uneasiness, discontent and impatience because that is the natural mind of human beings. But human beings have a deep wisdom and can cultivate it through detachment from their emotions. They can then be calm and pure in mind in any circumstance and any environment."

I couldn't reply to him. I thought that what he said was true and remembered that this is also the teaching of Zen. His words struck home to me, despite my anxieties, more deeply than anything I had previously heard or read.

Still I wanted to be like this old man and wondered how on earth I could get such a mind? I reflected that I had been unable to find the answer from any religion I had encountered in the past. At length I asked him again—

"Please tell me the difference between the mind of human beings and the mind of animals?"

He said—"Animals do sometimes feel anxious and an animal can get angry when it is ill or afraid. That is the natural mind of animals and, although we also have that mind, we don't need to indulge it. But to laugh and feel peaceful in spite of difficulties and danger and to love the one who has injured you requires training. Only through training can we become fully human. This teaching was given to me so many times in my childhood. My father was a realized person who taught me that the essential training of religion is training to control the mind. With such training, your mind will be peaceful and you won't have anxiety. If you are arrested then what has happened reflects your own attitude. Why have I been arrested?" He laughed. "My name was so bad that I was arrested."

For a few days I asked no more questions but simply tried to follow his practices. Although I couldn't understand his meditation at that time I found that just being with him and chanting his prayers and *mantras* made me feel calm and peaceful. Gradually I did learn his meditation and compared it with the meditation of Zen, Tibetan Buddhism and Indian Yoga. I thought how wonderful it would be if I also could learn to meet any situation with a calm and tranquil mind. I wondered at times if meditation was the best way, but I had to admit to myself that at no time had I really devoted myself to meditation. A few days later I again asked the old man a question—

"What is the quickest way of attaining true humanity?"

He replied—"The best way is to have faith."

I said to him—"I have no faith, but I will pray to something or someone if you tell me to do so."

He said—"You don't need to pray. True faith is the wisdom which can accept everything with laughter, pleasure, and gratitude. If you have faith you don't reject anything. You are able to accept everything as God's teaching and so you can leave things to take their course. If you have this faith you will be tranquil."

I realized then that religions are all teachings which, in different ways, bring us to this mind of faith. The conclusion of all religions is the same—to reach the perfection of *satori* we must practice love. I wonder if my reader follows a religion, or if you have ever asked yourself seriously "What is God?" or "What is *satori*?" When I heard the old man using the words God, religion and love, it was as if he had struck deeply into my mind. I had had much contact with religious groups since childhood, but I had never sought them out voluntarily. In spite of all my chances I had never deliberately sought for God. At my father's funeral I had thought that religion was ridiculous. I refused to permit the monks to enter the house and threatened them with a sword! My mother cried for a week. At one time I had tried to cure my tuberculosis through religion because my father, who was devoted to Zen, urged me to do so. But these contacts were far from the intense desire of spiritual need. Although I knew all about the ways of the different religious sects, I had little idea what the name of God meant.

Because of my background I felt compelled to answer the old man's questions in a certain way. When he asked me—

"Have you ever sought God?"

I replied—"I have always thought of God but I cannot believe that he exists. In spite of much experience of religion I cannot tell you what God is. Please tell me the answer."

At that time I had a burning desire to know the answer because the old man made me feel that something incredibly precious was shining out of him. His complete purity and openness seemed to absorb everything in the world. I did not doubt that he was my teacher.

The gaol was small and dark; there was a small light burning in one corner. The old man bent slightly forwards as he sat there, talking quietly. He looked like God himself. He smiled at my questions and said—

"Do you expect me to explain God in words? I can't. In my youth I also pursued the same question. I intended to be a businessman and my youthful confidence was such that I thought I could explain God. People said that I had much force and intensity but, although I believed in God, I had no calmness of mind.

"With age and experience I came to see that my ideas about God were mistaken. To correct this condition we must be absolutely honest with ourselves and this is what I tried to do."

The old man's gentle teaching made me realize that I was really unaware of the realities of life. After this realization I was more and more able to accept everything which came to me with gratitude and to give with joy. This is the life of non-resistance and it led me to see that God permits me to live, protects me, provides for me, and loves me. I began to realize the real meaning of salvation and *satori*. I realized that I was saved from the beginning, am saved now, and will be saved in the future. I no longer wanted anything and so I could appreciate the value of everything. I was able to accept everything just as it is and to see that everything is already perfect. When I gained such a flexible mind, life became tremendously enjoyable.

The reason why I had not been able to understand God, and the reason why most people do not understand God, is because we try to know him intellectually. You must feel God with your whole being, not try to think him. I was deeply impressed by the teaching of the old man, but I could ask no more questions. The night was far advanced and we were both very tired. The next day he told me that he had come to feel something of God by knowing himself, and by having the humble mind of gratitude and acceptance. His manner was quiet and passive, yet what he said excited me more strongly than anything I had previously heard or read. That night I had great difficulty in finding sleep because my mind was full of longing and fell into disorder. Whenever I thought about God my mind became full of thoughts of "what" and "how" and I was overcome by my feelings. This was very different to the mind of *satori* which sees reality as it is.

The next day, my old friend ate only a little food. His long training had enabled him to live on very little and so he gave me half his meal. I could see that he did not look tired and was astonished at his vitality. He was far more lively and active than I! I said to him—"I want to know God—I tried to feel God in bed last night, but I could not."

He smiled and said—"So you want to change from an animal to a human being do you? Good!"

After some time he said—

"What you can feel is not God, but the mind of God."

I couldn't understand this but didn't ask any more questions just then. After lunch, he began to chant *mantra* as usual and now I could follow him easily. It is very difficult to understand any sacred writing in its original script and Arabic is said to be the most difficult language in the world. The old man's *Koran* was written in ancient Arabic but I remembered the basic teaching by writing down in Japanese what he read to me in English. Basically the *Koran* tells us that it is our duty to praise the virtue of God, that we should submit ourselves fully to his will and follow him, and that God is absolute love. After being with the old man I saw that I was far away from such a condition but wanted to change and become like him. Later I again asked him—

"What should I do to feel the mind of God?"

"To feel the mind of God is to feel true joy and to see reality as it is" he said.

I replied—"Is reality God's mind?"

"Yes" he said, "The Universe itself is God. The whole appearance is the mind of God and you can come to understand this through nature. Normally we see a tree as a tree and a stone as a stone. That is animal mind. You must learn to see the inner life of trees and stones and then you will realize that they are not what they seem, but God. Then you will feel that you are in Paradise even here in this gaol. Such a condition means that the eye of mind has opened. If you want to know the real God you must give up your own views and the God you have made yourself."

At that point he began to meditate again and I began to wonder about the God I had made myself. I realized with a shock that I had thought about God only when I was in trouble or difficulties. In gaol I had prayed eagerly because I wanted to find a way to be saved. I didn't really believe that God existed, yet I was asking him for something. I was praying only because there was nothing else I could do and I was praying to the God I had made myself. In normal life I had been totally unaware of God, but I had heard that people who believed in him were stronger. I wondered why? I had heard that God will give us power and that God is within. What is that God? My old friend and teacher had told me that I couldn't know God by thinking.

After supper, the old man asked—

"Do you want to know God?"
"Yes" I replied.
"There is no way of grasping God by means of the mind" he said. "I can't give you any explanation. Theology is learning, but faith is not. Reading books and listening to lectures is not enough. You can only come to know God by persistently living the right life. Depth of faith depends, finally, on God."

I asked him to explain about the right way of life. He said—

"There are many ways of purifying the mind and body and opening the eye of mind. What you must do is, firstly, laugh and have the mind of gratitude and, secondly, give up all your ideas about yourself."

I asked him—"Must I laugh always and have gratitude for everything?"

"Yes" he replied. "If we don't do these things we cannot know real joy. Only a person who lives with this mind can know and love God."

"Do you enjoy even the threat of death?" I asked him.

He said—"Yes I do! I may not be executed, but even if I am I want to die with human dignity. It is a mistake to feel anxious about things which are not certain; and it is especially useless to complain about things which are certain."

I wondered how I could have such calm composure even in such a terrible situation. If we can laugh under threat of execution then surely we can laugh at any time. The old man explained that the way is to always practice being pleasant to others and enjoy everything without trying to impose any conditions. Until we are in this state we must contrive to raise, improve and develop ourselves in every way.

In everyday life it is necessary to employ a dual approach to reality. What we can understand we should study and think about, but what we cannot understand we should keep an open mind. In *satori* the mind does not ask foolish questions and the most foolish question of all is "What is God?"

The old man said to me—

"When you are young, you may think that God is the universe, or that God is your own will. There are two fates: one is constructed by ourselves but the other is given. We can control our own fate to a large extent but the fate given by others contains something of the inevitable. When you realize this you come to accept everything meekly as God's gift. I feel that you have the wrong way of life. Allowing matters to take their own course is actually very positive. It means doing your utmost to the very end and then, when you can do no more, accepting God's will completely. When you know that you have done your best, you are not concerned with any reward. Then you can be calm. At the moment you are not alive. Have you never felt that you have life only as a privilege? To be permitted to live is to be given the most wonderful gift, to be protected and to be saved. Practice devoting yourself to the thought—'I am permitted to be alive.'"

As I listened to him my mind became clear and calm. I told him about it and he said that this extreme condition of mind is the religious mind. It is called *satori* in Buddhism and *samadhi* in Yoga.

Two months had passed and one night when I was in bed, I heard a lot of noise and the sound of rifle fire. The old man shook me and said—

"My comrades have come to save me, would you like to come?"

"Yes," I replied.

There seemed to be about thirty people in the raiding party and I ran off into the darkness with them, although I didn't know where they were going. When I think of this night now, it reminds me of a Western film at the cinema! By the next evening we reached their retreat and I stayed there one night. My old friend suggested to me that the best way of attaining my purpose of entering Central Asia was to join the religious mendicancy of Islam which was accepted throughout that huge region. He told me that one of his friends, who was head of an important Islamic sect, was currently staying in Ispahan and that I could go to him. Next day I said farewell to my old friend and left for Ispahan accompanied by two of the comrades. On the way, they explained to me about the old man. "His name is Hoseini-shi (teacher Hoseini)" they said, "and he is the head of Islam in Iran." Some time after the war I happened to see his picture

The Sacred in Gaol—The Teaching of Hoseini-shi

in the newspaper at the time of the civil disturbances in Iran under Prime Minister Mosadec. I tried to get Hoseini's address through the Embassy, but I could not. I wanted to tell him that at last I had been able to enter the spiritual life and that what he had taught me during those two months was still living in my heart. Nothing impressed me more as a young man than the serene teaching of Hoseini. Hoseini and Gandhi were the beloved teachers who opened my eyes to the genuine life of religion. For many years I longed for their company and found myself eagerly seeking for their books, but I always felt that simple gratitude was not enough. That is why I am recording here what Hoseini said.

"The movement of life within us is the movement of God. We cannot know God or life by thinking about it, nor can we see it, for what we see is only an appearance. The way to know God is to fulfill the condition that we must improve ourselves to the utmost, then God will appear."

In later years I was taught in Yoga that God is life and God is nature. I had felt I could grasp even the most profound truth from Hoseini because he was a man who had attained *satori* through Yoga. Religion does not mean being able to give logical explanations, or construct complex theories. It is rather to love the truth, to seek the truth and to practice the truth in your life. We must try to know God with our whole being.

This is the mind of being fully alive, that we should make water and air alive and bring life to all things including other people and ourselves. To bring things to life is faith. To give the body correct nutrition is faith, to have right breathing is faith and to make the best use of money is faith, for that means that we are bringing money alive. So, too, it is faith to make the best use of your own talents and to encourage others to do the best with theirs. We should not eat wrong food if we want to make our body alive, nor should we use our bodies unreasonably. To make the mind more alive we should not occupy it with trivial things. If you want the truth you don't need to know the answer to the question "What is God?" Just pray without rationalization, practice *Meiso Yoga* without theorizing, for you should not do these things with the attitude of seeking for something. We should pray that we may give up the sense of ownship of ideas and actions and practice *Zazen* in order to come to the unconditioned mind. If the mind is free it can become the mind of God. Making your mind empty means praying for God and not for yourself. When the mind is being emptied of thoughts of self in meditation, it is being purified.

When you are in trouble pray quietly and practice *Meiso Yoga* in the spirit—"If I were God, how would I think and act?" This visualization will help to arouse the mind of God in you. I have had cause to appreciate this valuable teaching many times and I would like to pass it on to others. It is the best way of conducting our lives, for real love means to devote yourself wholeheartedly to God. If you seek things for yourself it is not love, for love of what you want to get can easily become hate. Love without conditions is treasure indeed, but love with conditions is the seed of torture. The love of God goes on loving no matter what happens, for God doesn't have anything in his heart, neither linking nor disliking, enemy or friend. In God there is only love. That is *satori* mind—to love even if the result is against what you hoped for and even if there are difficulties, suffering and torture. When we compare the love of God with the love of human beings we can see that human love is but a pale shadow of the real thing. I cannot help feeling that it is an impertinence to use the word love for human emotions.

A sense of difficulty and agony of mind result from being opposed to someone or something. Are you waiting for an apology from someone? If so, you will have no harmony in your heart as long as you live. If you swallow your pride and apologize first, the gate of harmony will be opened. Animals cannot apologize: the mind of gratitude and the soul of apology means that you are approaching the fully human condition. If you can attain unconditional love, that is the very mind of God. In this state the true joy is given and the sunshine of peace will shine but such harmony means giving up all selfishness. Everyone today has a lot to say, but for God's sake we must abandon our viewpoints. Try only to feel gratitude to all and to accept everything as God's teaching. These principles are what Life has taught me and although you will find here what Hoseini or

Gandhi said, it is not really their teaching. I have made it my own by putting it into actual practice and that is Yoga. The teaching of Hoseini and Gandhi was, however, the beginning of my faith.

When I meet apparently insurmountable difficulties, I think of the time which I spent in gaol with Hoseini. The memory of Holy teachers is always the source of our greatest inspiration. I was taught by Hoseini about Islam and the relationship between Zoroastrianism and Judaism. He was also the person who first taught me about the Vedas and who gave me detailed explanations of the Yogic ascesis, or training method. Hoseini was also the teacher of some of Gandhi's closest friends and, although I have since accepted teachings from many other sources, I still remember clearly what these two great men taught me. When I was with Hoseini, my mind grasped the truth like lightning. I was really listening to every word he said. Even if others had received the same teaching they would not have understood it as I did. At that time I was very near to death and my mind was full of thoughts about being saved. I was seeking desperately for something, like a drowning man clutching at a straw. Also I was continuously chanting *mantra* and practicing meditation with him. Even though two people eat the same food, the effect may be quite different if one of them is meditating and praying. It is the same in the case of taking medicine or doing a job. As I had a good deal of knowledge about Yoga already, I could easily accept the concept of a step by step training. The first step is to purify and unify the body and mind by conscious effort and to attain to the mind of *Mushin*. The second is to expand the mind effortlessly into the infinite space of *satori*.

3. The Uses of Fear in Esoteric Religious Systems

The religious mendicants to whom Hoseini introduced me were called "curs" by the common people, but their correct name is the *Dervishes*. You might think that these wanderers were idealistic philosophers living a life of freedom. They never formed large groups and their general code of behavior was very pure and strict. All religious groups seek the true way in the beginning, but when they get power they tend to lose their initial purity. They are distorted and disordered by over-concern with material well-being and authoritarianism. They no longer provide a suitable means for the true seeker. Mohammed founded Islam as a way of returning to God. His religion was based on equality, love, service, and real spirituality, but, with the passing of the years, these ideals faded. The same is true in principle of all the major religions. This process always throws up groups of true seekers who break away from orthodoxy and return to the simple basic principles of the way. The religious mendicancy I met was such a group.

To regain purity of purpose they renounced social life and possessions. Living without any material security they devoted their lives to serving God without any conditions whatsoever. Their discipline included the control of desire, various forms of penitence, chanting and meditation. Their aim was to follow the teaching of the Prophet and to maintain their vows of poverty, chastity and obedience whilst living as wandering priests. This life style places special importance on willingness to accept all things as God's will, to live only on what is freely given and to abandon self-will. By accepting all things as divine teachings and consciously bearing all sufferings in a spirit of service, they hoped to draw near to the mind of God. Their precepts might be expressed as follows:

1. At all costs do without what is not given.
2. If you are denied, resist anger.
3. Never indulge in flattery to encourage the giver.
4. Do not buy your needs.
5. Accept all circumstances with gratitude and without complaint.

Like the first Buddhists, the mendicants went about serving society and receiving a share of its produce in return. They were not really beggers. Amongst the contemporaries of the Buddha, some went out with a bowl to receive offerings. So, they were called *Bhikkhus*, or "sharesmen," and they were full of ardent spiritual ambition.

The Uses of Fear in Esoteric Religious Systems / 151

The Character of the Dervishes: These seekers accept only the authority of God and oppose both civil and religious authority. In consequence, they have often suffered from persecution and have tended to become well-organized and secretive. By the control of desire and the practice of concentration many of their number developed supernormal powers and were held in some awe by the rest of the population. They obeyed the orders of their leaders unconditionally and had a strong sense of group identity. There were about thirty sects of these Sufistic wanderers and the one I joined emanated from *Bokara*, in Central Asia. All of them had this in common: that they sought the direct realization of God within.

The Conditions of Entry: After I had been introduced by my two comrades, I asked the Sheik, or head of the group if I could join them. I was told that all newcomers must serve a three-year probationary period. If their progress was not satisfactory during that time then they were not accepted. The probation was a period of training with almost military discipline to prepare the newcomer for renunciation of self and total reliance upon God.

1. In the first year they practiced prayer in order to root out selfishness and to learn to esteem others. Sheik said that the time comes when you can love, value, and respect everyone. When you can also see yourself in this way, you can take the next step. If you fall away from the path in the slightest particular, you must begin the first year once again.

2. The second year's training was passed in service of God. This meant neither prayer nor chanting, but the practice of total acceptance and gratitude. The aim was to wean the mind away from selfish discrimination and even from liking and disliking. No feelings of discontent or reluctance were admissible, nor any negative emotions, such as hate or guilt. When the mind had become established in affirmative thinking and was always calm and peaceful, the next stage was open.

3. The third year was devoted to concentration practice, self-control and detachment. Throughout this year, silence was strictly observed, including silent chanting. Breathing exercises and sitting practice were also carried out.

Sheik explained all this to me and taught me as follows:
"We intend to find God within and, for that we need to be empty in mind and body. The empty mind is the mind without the slightest attachment, whilst the empty body is healthy and without abnormality. Illness and mental attachments in the form of theories and illusions hinder us in our purpose. Our energies are spent uselessly in fighting to control the mind. Yet our failure is only the result of a wrong way of life and not the result of any inherent weakness. So we have to learn to make the best use of all our difficulties in order to purify and develop ourselves. To know God, it is necessary to heal yourself. That is why we do service, meditation and prayer. Why don't you try it?"

I could not fault his explanation and reflected that it agreed with all that Hoseini had said about living the right life. However I had a difficult problem to resolve. My desire to join the group was compromised to some extent by my obligation to fulfill my mission as a spy. I did not feel I could undertake the spiritual life with complete honesty. I thought about the matter for a few days but I could see no other way of entering Central and Southern Asia. Finally I went to Sheik and explained that I could not be sure if I was fully serious about beginning the spiritual life. I asked him if I could join them for a trial period of one month. Sheik laughed and said "Is that so? Very well, please try." He asked me to undertake a certain discipline. I was to try to manage on only three hours sleep, to practice fasting, and to chant for at least fifteen hours a day. The *mantra* I was to use was *Atsuraho Acrabu*. I asked Sheik if there was any difference between this discipline and the practice of Yogins in India? He replied that all disciplines originally came from Yoga and that this was also true of Islam. What he had asked me to do was to carry out Yoga in the context of Islamic religious beliefs.

I had previously tried a little Yoga training in India, but it was not

The Uses of Fear in Esoteric Religious Systems / 153

fully intensive. This was the first time I had undertaken full spiritual discipline and the next ten days were very hard indeed. The most difficult thing was to repeat the *mantra* continuously. When I was with Hoseini in gaol I thought that simply repeating the name of God was rather pointless, although I accepted that it was one of the ways of faith. I still felt that it was foolish, but I continued nevertheless. But even though I chanted I thought of other things and concentration eluded me. Then, suddenly, the realization of God hit me like a physical blow and I knew that what I was doing was the right discipline for me at that time. When the first day ended I was exhausted and slept deeply. On the second day everything in me refused to continue, but nevertheless I persevered. It was probably much more difficult because I was also fasting. Anyway my pride drove me on and I completed the second day. On the third day, my throat was swollen and painful and I could only whisper and croak. I tried hard for the next nineteen days. My previous training stood me in good stead and I had the experience of forgetting everything. After that the Sufi who had been made responsible for me told me to do sitting practice, like *Zazen*. I do not remember whether I fasted or not. Anyway I practiced detachment from thought for five days and, meanwhile, he taught me the methods of gazing at one point and counting the breaths.

The human mind feels light and airy under these conditions and I experienced no difficulty during those five days. The biggest difference I noticed between the practice of this meditation and that of Japanese Zen was that, by this way, it was easier to unify the mind and to attain even greater stability. It was a severe training in the unification of consciousness and I felt that I had attained *Mushin*, or empty mind. The next five days were to lead me to the opening of the "eye of the mind." I was instructed to stare at the face of Sheik for a while and then I was blindfolded when he gave the signal. A little later, the blindfold was removed and I saw Sheik's face again. During the time I was blindfolded, I retained the image of his face in my mind. I remembered that I had seen Yogins doing a similar thing by opening and closing their eyes. For five days I continued this practice and, on the fifth day, I found that I could visualize

Sheik's face with great clarity at any time.

The Burning Stick Attached to the Body: I was told that, in the course of the next ten days, my progress would be examined. I wondered what on earth they would do to me. The Sufi explained that, in order to see if my mind was really in the state of *Mushin* they would either cut me, or attach a smoldering stick to my body. Genuine *Mushin* is a state in which the self has been completely renounced but what people think is *Mushin* can be a form of self-indulgence. If it is genuine, you do not feel physical pain. I was very much afraid I might feel pain and lacked confidence. Even if I had the real *Mushin* I thought I might nevertheless feel the burning stick. The more I thought about it, the stronger my fear became. The Sufi saw my discomfort and told me not to worry. He said that, in a few days time, I would realize that anyone can do it.

I had previously experienced burning the body without feeling pain. In Manchuria, there was a *Nichiren* sect which used a candle flame to burn the arms. The flame was very small and was brought close to the arm as you were chanting. If you chanted fiercely and with strong concentration, you could endure the heat. Nevertheless, I afterwards suffered from painful blisters for a few weeks. I think my fear of the burning stick was quite natural in the circumstances. Then the training began. On the first day there were six people including myself. We were shown how to move our bodies, adjust our breathing and concentrate our consciousness. At night we stared at the flame of a candle and we were each given a rosary for chanting. As we chanted we moved the beads from left to right.

At first, my mind was relaxed, but I forced myself to concentrate. After a few hours, I found myself chanting like a machine, for my mouth was moving independently. I wondered if I had attained the unconditioned state. Certainly, I was almost completely detached from thoughts and I felt that, not only my head, but my whole body was very light and floating, like a sleepwalker. When the others entered into *satori* they stood up and began to dance. They seemed to me to be crazy, but they were quite indifferent to others. As for me, I was still very concerned about time and the opinion of other people and could not gain the same condition.

On the second day, I felt that I was becoming more and more absorbed. I began to realize the true reason for chanting. The chanting had become a completely reflex action and I forgot about hunger for hours on end. Time passed very quickly and I did not notice that it had become dark. Eventually someone patted me on the shoulder and told me it was suppertime and then time-consciousness returned. It seemed to me that we had only just finished the previous meal and I wondered where the intervening time had gone. I thought that this might be *satori*. After supper my mind remained unsettled, however, and I continued to be aware of time. I again experienced a strong reluctance to practice. During the third day, I tried to attain *satori* but it was difficult and I felt irritated. Later in the morning I was able to enter into *satori* for about two hours. At that stage I was the only person who was eating, since the others were all fasting in preparation for the experience of the burning stick.

The Experience of the Burning Stick: It became evident that I was to be excluded from the experience on that occasion but I was still very anxious. At night a charcoal fire was made and a metal rod was heated. One man handled the bellows and the charcoal became white hot. The others seemed to me to be in deep *satori*. At ten o'clock, Sheik came with a sword and chains. He gave the chains to two people and they began to lash themselves. They hit themselves so severely that they bled copiously from wounds all over their bodies. The rest began to chant rapidly in order to stimulate the two even more.

I forgot to chant and just sat there watching them. Sheik went to the fire and withdrew the metal rod which was glowing red. When I realized what he was about to do I began to vomit. Sheik handed the rod to a man and he began to touch it to his body at random. The smell in that place was like dried cuttlefish! My attention was riveted to the scene and I was filled with astonishment. Another man took the sword and began to cut himself. He made deep cuts and the blood gushed out. They seemed like a crowd of demented demons and even those who were observing became half-crazy and chanted incessantly. I, too, began to chant, being unaware of what I was doing. The words just came out of my mouth automatically. Suddenly, Sheik screamed and four men fainted and fell down on the floor. Soon after that, I lost consciousness as well.

When I awoke, morning had come. The four men were sleeping besides me. I examined them and found that they were in a deep, almost drugged, sleep and were not dead. I removed the blankets and looked at their bodies. They were full of cuts, burns and wounds and were in very bad shape. The one who had burnt himself was in the worst condition. Strangely enough he did not have the inflammation and other symptoms which normally accompany burns. Olive oil had been applied to all the blisters. I lay down again and wondered if I could undergo such an experience. They had suffered no serious harm because they were genuinely absorbed in *satori*. I reflected that, on the previous night, my condition might have been described as "half-*satori*." On the whole, I felt that it would be wiser to stop. As I thought about it all, I fell asleep. Perhaps two hours passed before my companion awakened me. "Sheik is calling you" he said, and I experienced fear when I wondered what he might ask me to do today. I came to his tent trembling and, seeing my condition, he smiled and said:

"Well, what do you say now? You can do it easily if you are in *satori* for you will have lost all physical sensation as well as becoming detached from thought and emotion. It means that you will have become released from the self. Today we are going to do the last *satori* training through the body. Your four companions will sleep until tomorrow and, even though they have many cuts and burns, their bodies will be healed by the time they awake. You may find this difficult to believe, but you will see for yourself that it is so. When we are burnt in our normal state of mind, we have the thought "I am burnt" and this makes it worse. When we do not realize that we have been injured the pain is slight. As soon as we become aware of the injury the mind becomes disordered and the pain begins. Did you know that?"

I replied:

"No, I didn't know. However, I am very disturbed by my experi-

The Uses of Fear in Esoteric Religious Systems / 157

ences last night and I think it would be wisest for me to end my probation. I feel that I cannot attain *satori* unless I can practice for the full three years." Sheik gazed into my eyes and said:
"If you wish to you can stop, but if you do I cannot allow you to enter our sect again. I am not trying to coerce you, but we can only accept those who have a deep resolve to train. The others are only human, you know. You can do what they did, so don't be afraid. If you will only try you will find it easy, but you cannot know this merely by discussion. Even if you want to stop I recommend you to undergo this experience today. You may gain some deep wisdom even though you subsequently leave our sect. Even if you feel that you cannot take the full experience again, I suggest that you should at least practice sitting concentration for another five days in order to open yourself fully to *satori*."

The Fateful Experience: After hearing what Sheik said, I decided to accept his advice. I resolved to continue the discipline in some form even if I did not undergo the complete thing. As I left his presence, Sheik asked me not to wake the other disciples. When I returned later in the day, however, the one who had burnt himself and the one who had beaten himself with the chain were awake. They appeared to be absent-minded and, when I asked about their wounds, they did not reply. One of them removed his garment and I could see that only slight red marks remained. "Did you feel any pain?" I asked, but he only shook his head.

I still felt disinclined to repeat the training because of my fear. On the following day, the other three disciples appeared and urged me to continue concentration practice and fasting. At that time, I felt I could not join them again, but once I began to practice, I entered quickly into deep meditation. It was as if all my previous training was synthesized and my mind became very still and calm. I noticed neither the passage of time nor a feeling of hunger. The days passed quickly and my absorption became ever deeper. I could see, hear, and understand everything, but I was not interested in analyzing my experience. It was so fascinating that I had no wish to stop. It was the experience of *satori*.

On the fifth day, the charcoal fire was lit again and the iron rod was heated. I had a vague idea that I might be able to take part in this strange ceremony tonight. Soon the sounds of a drum and a bell were heard and the atmosphere became truely electric. It is very difficult to convey the feeling in words, but it arose from a combination of music, prayer, and movement and it produced a sense of ecstasy. Many hours passed and I began to have the strange feeling that I was being controlled by some benevolent, external power. I lost the ability to stand aside from the total situation. The disciples danced and chanted *mantra*, casting exotic silhouettes on the walls by the light of the fire. Soon I too began to dance, moved by a will which was not my own, for I could not, and did not want to, regain normal consciousness at that time.

Then the atmosphere changed and I glanced back to see Sheik gazing at me. Just then, one of the dancers came to the fire and withdrew the heated rod. Although I was in a dream-like state, I clearly observed what he did. He began to touch his body with the red-hot rod and, once again, I smelt burning flesh. Others followed, one by one, and did the same. I still doubted if it were possible for me to copy them, but gradually my doubts evaporated in that ecstatic atmosphere. Suddenly I found myself besides the fire, taking hold of the rod. I was full of fear, but the power which controlled me, as I stood there chanting the *mantra*, bade me carry on.

Although I definitely touched myself, I felt nothing. It was like acting in a dream, yet I was able to observe myself clearly and objectively. The first touch miraculously changed my fear into excitement and stimulated me to do it again and again. Soon, I was hitting my body at random. It could be described as the insanity of a clear and lucid consciousness. I lost count of the number of times I touched myself and, shortly afterwards, I lost consciousness completely.

It was the afternoon of the next day but one before I awoke, or so I was told afterwards. Although I had opened my eyes, I still felt that I was in a dream, yet my mind was able to witness all events. At the same time, I felt refreshed, just as you do after experiencing strong excitement. My mind ranged over the events of the previous days. I knew that I had burnt myself, yet I also knew that it was not I who had willed it. I began to doubt if I had really done it, for my mind would not accept such a thing. For a while I slept again and I was told later that I slept longer than any of the others. The next time I awoke, I was no longer in the dream-like state, but had returned to a very clear and more normal state of consciousness. Suddenly I remembered the burns and sat up swiftly to look at my body. There were only slight discolorations where the burns had been, surrounded by a faint redness. I moved, but although my skin felt a little strange, my body as a whole felt quite normal. I touched the places where the burns had been, but there was no soreness.

At that moment, Sheik returned to me and said:

"So, you're awake again! You slept long because I gave you a sleeping draught when you first opened your eyes. It was still too early for you to wake up because your blisters were not then healed. Your consciousness is not yet fully based upon *satori* and your physical condition would have become worse. Whilst you slept your mind was stable and your body could work in the very highest condition. Deep sleep can heal many illnesses which would be far more difficult to disperse when the mind is changeable and unstable. That's why animals instinctively sleep when they are ill, or injured. Think about this deeply, try to understand why the mind becomes unstable and see what it is that you should do. It is very difficult to be genuine."

I thought about his words a great deal. I had had the experience of deep *satori*, for which I was profoundly grateful. Although I had come to the sect with a strictly non-spiritual purpose, what I had experienced enabled me to realize the true meaning of religious practice.

The Importance of Learning through the Body: My experiences affected me very deeply during the days and weeks that followed. I realized that doing is so much more important than knowing. It was a rare and wonderful opportunity for me and opened my eyes to many things. After the teaching of Hoseini, I had experienced meditation and *satori*, but I now feel that they were not quite the real thing. Although I had experienced the total concentration of body and mind, the change in my state of consciousness was not under my own control. I did it only with the help of external discipline and a very favorable atmosphere. Only when we can unify body and mind at will and freely attain *satori* at any time, is it the real thing. Nevertheless, this experience was a great step forwards because in all my later training I knew precisely what I was seeking to attain.

I hope that as a result of reading this book, others will be able to distinguish more accurately between the real and the false in spiritual training and spiritual experience. I want to emphasize the fact that no-one can attain *satori* without dedicated training and that there are well-tried ways and methods. Above all, the training must be followed step by step. Only then can consciousness attain freedom and full autonomy.

Glossary

Asanas (Sc.)   The postures of Yoga which demonstrate one-pointed concentration, physically.

Astanga Yoga (Sc.)   The Yoga of eight "limbs," or stages, taught by *Patanjali*.

Atman (Sc.)   The real self, or principle of consciousness. Thatr portion of universal consciousness which is incarnated in the individual.

Bhakti Yoga (Sc.)   The Yoga of self-effacement through love and devotion to God.

Bodhisattva (Sc.)   The ideal state of *Mahayana* Buddhism in which human nature is completely spiritualized. *Bosatsu* (J.)

Bosatsu (J.)   see *Bodhisattva*.

Brahman (Sc.)   The God of the Aryans. See Brahmanism.

Brahmanism (Sc.)   The ancient religion of the Aryans which is one of the main elements in the modern Indian amalgam of religions known as Hinduism.

Budo (J.)   A collective term for all the arts which have been raised to the level of spiritual disciplines. In Japan, Budo includes all the martial arts, for religion touched them and turned them into ways of the spirit.

Bussho (J.)   The faculty of real understanding which, with *Hannya*, forms what is termed human wisdom.

Danjiki (J.)   Mental fasting which, through the training of not eating, leads to *Mu*-Mind.

Danshari (J.)   The enlightened practice of fasting extended to all human behavior, literally, the cutting off of bad habits.

Dharana (Sc.)	Concentration practice. In Japanese; *Isshin*. *Isshin* leads to *Mushin*.
Dhyana (Sc.)	Unity. *Dharana* is concentration; *Dhyana* is release. *Dharana* is one-pointed unity and *Dhyana* is total, universal unity.
Dozen (J.)	Movement performed with a heightened awareness: hence mobile meditation and utmost stability.
Gyo (J.)	To use every circumstance and every activity as training. Exercise is *Gyo* only when it is done with awareness of its spiritual purpose: e.g. *Zengyo*.
Hannya (J.)	The natural wisdom which is rooted in the structure of living cells.
Hara (J.)	The lower abdominal center of the nervous system and the musculature; the physical and emotional center of gravity of the body responsible for stability and balance. Known as *Uddiyana* in India, it was called *T'an T'ien* in China and this was transliterated into Japanese as *Tanden*.
Hatha Yoga (Sc.)	Yoga derived from *Raja* Yoga which places most emphasis on physical disciplines.
Hoetsu (J.)	Enlightenment, or pure religious ecstasy.
Jnana (Sc.)	The Yoga of philosophical analysis.
Karma Yoga (Sc.)	The Yoga of service and action.
Kensho (J.)	The state in which man manifests his full value, the obverse of *satori*.
Ki (J.)	See *Prana*.
Kinen (J.)	Literally, "the practice of the praying mind." Analogous in some ways to *Bhakti* Yoga.
Kriya Yoga (Sc.)	The Yoga of techniques for purifying mind and body.
Kumbhaka (Sc.)	Retention of the breath.

Kundalini Yoga (Sc.)	The Yoga which raises the basic sexual-energy and uses it to burn away the barries to universal consciousness.
Mahayana (Sc.)	The great school of Northern Buddhism which gave rise to the Zen and *Shingon* sects.
Mantra Yoga (Sc.)	The Yoga of chanting and magic.
Meiso (J.)	Meditation in the usually accepted sense of sitting and concentration practice.
Meiso Yoga (J.)	A higher level of consciousness reached as a result of regarding the whole of life as training. It is the true meditation.
Mikkyo (J.)	The esoteric religious tradition of Buddhism.
Mu (J.)	Consciousness freed from the limitations of contingent thought has the quality of emptiness. Being empty of all restriction, it is open to all meaning. This is the state of *Mu*.
Mudra (Sc.)	Static or mobile postures, mainly of the hands, which are often used with *mantra*.
Nirvana (Sc.)	See *Satori*.
Niyama (Sc.)	The rules of personal morality in Yoga.
Okidō (J.)	The Way of Oki. A *Dō* is a complete life-style which includes religion, philosophy and science.
Patanjali (Sc.)	The author of the Yoga Sutra who was the first to organize Yogic knowledge into a coherent system.
Prana (Sc.)	The universal energy which man is sometimes permitted to conduct. Called *Ki* in Japanese.
Pranayama (Sc.)	Yogic breathing exercises aimed at raising and controlling the movement of *Prana*.
Pratyahara (Sc.)	Withdrawal of the senses.
Raja Yoga (Sc.)	The Yoga which emphasizes mental discipline and meditation.

Reikan (J.) — Literally "soul-feeling" or intuition.

Samadhi (Sc.) — See *Satori*.

Samkhya (Sc.) — One of the most ancient schools of Indian philosophy.

Samon (Sc.) — The ancient fathers of Yoga and followers of the indigenous religion of the Indus valley. *Samon:* means "freedom."

Samurai (J.) — The warriors of medieval Japan whose training methods and code of honor have done much in shaping modern martial arts. See *Budo*.

Sanmitsu (J.) — Unity of three; in Yoga, the unity of body, mind and breath.

Satori (J.) — The fundamental spiritual experience of oneness, or union, which is given by the truth of human nature but colored by religious beliefs. In India it is called *Samadhi* or *Nirvana* but is known by many other names throughout the world.

Sennin (J.) — The Japanese ascetics of the mountains.

Shakuhachi (J.) — A traditional Japanese musical instrument. An end-blown bamboo flute on which is played the music of meditation.

Shorinji Kemyo (J.) — A form of unarmed self-defense which is part of *Budo*.

Shuseiho (J.) — The special Corrective Exercises of Okidō.

Tai Chi Ch'uan (Ch.) — A Chinese form of *Dozen*, or mobile meditation. In Japanese *Tai Kyoku Ken*.

Tanden (J.) — See *Hara*.

T'an T'ien (Ch.) — See *Hara*.

Tapas (Sc.) — The inner fire or spiritual aspiration.

Uddiyana (Sc.) — See *Hara*.

Glossary / 165

Veda (Sc.)	The ancient scriptures first introduced into India by the Aryans about 2000–1500 B.C.
Vedanta (Sc.)	A later school of Indian philosophy founded by *Sankarachaya*. *Vedanta* means "the completion of the *Vedas*."
Yama (Sc.)	The universal moral laws.
Yogasanas (Sc.)	See *Asanas*.
Zanmei (J.)	The process leading to *satori*.
Zazen (J.)	Formal sitting practice in Zen Buddhism aimed at gaining stability of mind and body.
Zen (J.)	A sect within the *Mahayana* tradition of Buddhism which originated in China and reached its highest development in Japan. The three main Zen sects are *Rinzai, Soto,* and *Obaku*.
Zengyo (J.)	Zen training.

Ch. = Chinese   J. = Japanese   Sc. = Sanscrit

List of Okidō Address

ENGLAND

DAVID BRADSHAW
13c., Middle Way, Lewes, England
Tel. 07916-77177

GEOF D'ARCY
17, Prestwick Close, West Town Lane, Brislington, Bristol., England

DAVID GRIFFITHS
65, Gwili Terrace, Mayhill, Swansea, Wales, G.B.
Tel. 53190

FRANCE

ASSOCIATION FRANCAISE D'OKIDO
Place 50, 50, rue du Faubourg St. Dennis, Paris, France
Tel. 700-2054

JEAN SOUBERBIELLE
52, Rue de Charonne, 75011 Paris, France
Tel. 700-2054

JAPAN

OKI YOGA DŌJŌ
450-1 Sawachi, Mishima-Shi, Shizuoka-ken, Japan
Tel. 0559-86-5655

SHIMOKITAZAWA DŌJŌ
2-25-19, Daizawa Setagaya-ku, Tokyo, Japan
Tel. 03-422-0920

OSAKA DŌJŌ
3-27, Tosaboridori, Nishi-ku, Osaka, Japan
Tel. 06-441-3664

These are the main Dōjōs only:

NORTH AMERICA BLAKE GOULD, OKIDŌ GUILD OF AMERICA
373, Commonwealth Ave, Boston, Mass. 02115, U.S.A.
Tel. 617—262—1525

YUKIKO IINO
167 West 85th Street, New York, N.Y. 10024, U.S.A.
Tel. 212-873-4310

KANJITSU IIJIMA, DHARMA YOGA CHURCH INSTITUTE
10824 Baskel Ave, Granada Hills, Calif. 91344, U.S.A.

SOUTH AFRICA LYN DORFLING
141, Second Ave, Edenvale, TVL., South Africa

SOUTH AMERICA NOBU GOI
Rue Visconde, Do Rio Brano 828, Curitiba, Parana, Brazil

YUKIO AKIMOTO, DALMA LTDA.
Rua Cons. Furtado, 298–308, Liberdade, Sao Paulo, Brazil

KIYOAKI OKUHATA
Casilla Correo, 1127 Asunision, Paraguay

SWITZERLAND JEAN ROFIDAL
14, Rue des Delices, Geneve, Switzerland
Tel. 45-02-30

Index

abdominal breathing 56
abnormality 57
acceptance 37
acid food 66
acupuncture 135
adjusting breath 100
adjusting posture 100
adrenalin 93
Akarma 73
alkaline foods 63
Anahata 101
Anahata Tanani 101
anal sphincter muscle 100, 104
Analects of Confucius, the 19
animal protein 65
Anitara Yoga 117
anjinryume 47
anus 54
apperception 107
Aquinas, Thomas 82
Ananyakas 24
ardor 45, 46
Aryan 22–24
asanas 19, 21, 26, 32, 42, 48, 52, 53, 59, 76, 79, 109, 131
asceticism 33
Astanga Yoga 21
Atharva Veda 24
atheistic dualism 30
Atman 25, 29, 95, 102, 117, 119
Atsuraho Acrabu 152
attachment 94, 119
authoritarianism 150
autonomic nervous system 17, 78, 96
Awaking Vow 128
awareness 67, 125

bacilli 65
bad blood circulation 66
balance 53
balanced breathing 78
Bhagavad Gita 28
Bhakti 22, 81
Bhakti Yoga 21, 31, 32, 103, 120
Bhikkhus 150
blood circulation 131
blood poisoning 76
Bodhisattva 31
Bodhisattva ideal 19
body fluids 94
body-mind organism 119
Bokara 151
Bosatsu 31
Brahma 23
Brahman 23, 25, 29, 95, 102, 117, 119
Brahmanas 24
Brahmanism 23–26, 33
Brahmanistic Yoga 24
Brahmins 26
breath retention 78
breathing exercises 76
buckwheat noodles 135
Buddha, the 8, 13, 15, 16, 18, 25, 26, 28, 33, 45, 51, 72, 81, 84, 88, 94, 99, 103, 106, 120, 125, 140, 150
Buddhism 25, 26, 28, 33, 43, 73, 81, 119, 138, 141, 146
buppo 57
Bussho 10, 17, 37, 114

calcium 63
calm mind 92
calming hormone 56

170 / INDEX

calmness 45
cancer 64, 68, 75, 83, 106
celibracy 71
cerebral cortex 89, 95, 97, 98
Ch'an 103
Ch'an Buddhism 82
Chakras 63, 86, 101, 102
Chang-Tzu 60
Choshinho 100
Chosokuho 100
Christ, the 8, 13, 51, 72, 88, 120, 125, 140
Christian meditation 16
Christianity 13, 33, 43, 74, 81, 115
chronic fatigue 53
chronic illness 53, 75
chronic tiredness 57
chronicity 75
cleanliness 37, 45
Cleaning Vow 130
coexistence 87
cold baths 76
commonality of interest 121
concentration 26, 54, 79, 90–92, 99, 101
concentration practice 16
conscionsness 89, 90
Confucius 46
contagious disease 75
contemplation 33
continence 44
contraction 103
coprosperity 87
correct nutrition 147
corrective exercises 58, 77, 132
corpulency 75
cortex 17
criminal acts 96
cure-alls 40

Daimoku 102
Dainichi Nyorai 117
Dakurita 101

Danjiki 74, 75
Danshari 70–72, 96
deep peace 106
Dervishes 33, 34, 149, 151
detachment 16, 30, 42, 86, 88, 92, 129, 136
Dharana 26, 42, 81, 90, 91, 93, 99, 101, 103, 107, 109, 115
Dhyana 26, 42, 81, 90, 101, 103, 104, 107–109
diabetes 75
diaphragm 93
diseases of civilization 64
disunity 88
disunity of self 123
disunity of society 123
Dokkyo 130
Dōjō 19, 36, 49, 58, 67–71, 76, 78, 85, 87, 111, 127, 131, 132
Dōjō life 67
Dōzen 49, 54, 56, 105, 106
Dravidian 23

easy pose 100
effective relaxation 109
electrical potential 95
emotional stability 54
emptiness 25, 31
empty mind 100
end-gaining 36
enema 76
Enlightenment 9, 15, 18–21, 26, 43, 58, 72, 81, 90, 114, 116, 120, 125
enzymes 59, 63
Epicurus 44
erect posture 50
esoteric religion 125
esoteric sects 84
Etsudo 124
evacuation 76
evolutionary changes 98
exercise 37

exhalation 78, 112
exoteric sects 84
expansion 103
eye of the mind 153

faith 83, 106
fasting 27, 33, 69, 71–73, 75, 76
fatigue 52
fear 52
fermentation 64
festering 76
Five Precepts 43
flexibility 27
flower arranging 135
folk religion 82
freedom 33, 37, 116
fruit wine 63

gassho 68, 128, 130
Gedatsu 108
gentle massage 112
good and evil 69
good breathing 49
good diet 37
gratitude 67
gratitude in work 124
Greek philosophy 44
Gudoshin 106

Hannya 17, 118, 119
Hannya Shinkyo 78, 130
happiness 106
Happomoku 93
Hara 7, 16, 17, 20, 53–57, 76, 78, 79, 86, 88, 89, 93–96, 98, 100–102, 104, 105, 109, 110, 112, 113, 130, 131
Hara breathing 55
Hara power 93
harmony and balance 129
Hatha Yoga 21, 22, 31, 32, 117
health 70
heart disease 75

Heart Sutra 78
Hinayama 81
Hinduism 28
Hoetsu 9, 125
Hoseini-shi 146, 147, 149, 153
Hua Yen sect 5
human dignity 145
Hwa Yen 60
hypertensions 75

immanence 30
immutability 30
independence 27
Indian Ashrams 50
Indian meditation 16
Indian Yoga 18, 20, 33, 41, 51, 53, 87, 92, 141
individual training 134
individuality 30
inhalation 79
insight meditation 16
inspiration 118
insurmountable difficulties 149
integration 103
integrity 45, 69
intellectual ability 97
internal organ 50
internal resonance 79
intuition 118
inverted postures 53
Ishvara 30
Islam 13, 33, 74, 102, 138, 146, 149, 150, 152
Islamic meditation 16
Isshin 93, 107

Jainism 25, 26, 28, 33
Japanese character 116
Japanese meditation 16
Japanese sung poetry 135
Jnana Yoga 21, 22, 31
Jodo Shin-shu 32, 34
Judaism 33, 43, 74, 149

Kapila 30
Karma 81, 114, 116, 117
Karma Yoga 21, 32, 103, 120–122, 124
Karmic inheritance 91
Karmic relationships 83
Kataka Upanisad 29
Katas 99
Katha Upanisad 28, 117
Kegon 5, 60
Kenshin 115
Kensho 9, 106, 115
Ki 39, 59, 61, 77, 99
Kido 123
Kinen 58, 92, 106, 114, 115
Koran 144
Kriya Yoga 32
Ksatreyas 26
Kūkai 85, 117
Kumbhaka 78, 79, 99, 112
Kundalini Yoga 102
Kuriya 117
Kyokaho 132, 133

labor movements 122
Lao-Tzu 60, 72, 73
laughing exercises 134
Life-Force, the 14, 34, 35, 42, 47, 86, 113, 114, 117
life science 17
logical system 87
Lotus sects 31

macrobiotic food 67
Mahabharata 28
Mahayana 81
Mahayama Buddhism 119
Mahatma Gandhi 8, 18, 22, 25–27, 45, 103, 138, 147, 149
Mahavira 25
Manipuraka 63
mantra 85, 101, 102, 115–117, 139, 141, 143, 149, 152, 153

Mantra Yoga 32, 133
Marathon and cold bath 131
Martial Arts 40, 58, 77, 99, 108, 111, 133, 135
massage 135
material well-being 150
meditation 26, 27, 74, 118
meditation exercise 135
meditation practice 100
meditation training 104
Meiso 16, 96
Meiso Yoga 8–10, 16, 20, 25, 29, 37, 43, 45, 51, 58, 61, 99, 104, 106, 110, 118–120, 127, 147, 148
Mencius 46
mental detachment 72
merging with work 124
Mikkyo 72, 125
Mimasa 29
mind training 136
Miroku 16
Miso 64
miso soup 134
Mundra 130
mnemonics 97
mobile Zen 105
Mohenjo Dharo 22, 23, 52
moral corruption 81
Moses 43
Mozart, Wolfgang 33
Mu mind 25, 42, 135
Mumonkan 7
Mushin 88, 92, 93, 101, 102, 106–108, 114, 119, 122, 124, 149, 153, 154
Mushinho 100
Mushoku 74, 75

Nagajuna 31
Nashikagura Dharishita 101
Natas 26
natural abdominal breathing 96
natural balance 42, 60, 109, 112

natural condition 87
natural food 69
natural gratitude 98
natural heritage 98
natural hot-spring bath 135
natural rhythm 112
natural wisdom 77, 114
Nembutsu 102, 137
Nenriki 91
neurosis 86, 88
Nichiren 117, 154
Nirvana 24, 73, 114
Niyama 26, 42, 45, 47, 48
no intoxicants 44
non-anger 44
non-attachment 37, 92, 106
non-coveting 44
non-exaggeration 44
noṇ-lying 44
non-resentment 44
non-resistance 143
non-slandering 44
non-stealing 44
non-violence 44
Nyaya 30

Okidō 6, 16, 19, 28, 31, 32, 36, 39, 41, 49, 51, 53, 58, 77, 87, 104, 122, 128, 132
Okidō Dōjō 19, 86, 127
oneness 42
optimism 45
optimum physical condition 105
optimum state 95
Oriental philosophy 59
Oriental therapies 41
Ottma Daisojo 8
over-eating 96

palsy 75
Paradise 144
parasympathetic nervous system 92
Patanjali 21, 30, 31, 40, 42, 43, 45

patting 112
penitence 125
physical ability 73
physical distortions 20
physical power 89
physical strengthening exercises 109
physical training 83
pleasure in work 123
pose of adept 100
positive mind 115
practical exercises 83, 88
practical wisdom 95
Prakrti 29
Prana 26, 39, 59, 77, 86, 99
Pranayama 19, 21, 26, 42, 49, 59, 60, 61, 77, 79
Pratyahara 26, 42, 79, 80, 90, 107
prejudice 119
Prophet, the 150
Prophet Mohammed 8, 13, 33, 72, 150
protein 63
purification 20
Puritan mentality 122
Purusa 29
pyelitis 75

Raja Yoga 21, 22, 26, 31, 32, 120
rational mind 119
rationality 85, 119
rading 87
reflective meditation 16
Reikan 118, 119
relaxation 96, 103, 112
release 103
religion 27
religious ecstacy 43
religious language 129
reluctance 88, 91, 125, 151
renunciation 46
restlessness 86, 89
retirement 94
revelation 115

174 / INDEX

Rig Veda 24
right breathing 147
right diet 49, 77
Rinzai Zen 16, 91, 116
Rodin 15
Rodo 122

Sacred, the 9, 14, 30, 37, 48
sacred writing 84
salvation 143
Sama Veda 24
Samadhi 26, 42, 81, 146
Samkhya 21, 29, 30
Samkhya Yoga 5, 30
Samon 15, 23, 26, 27, 70
samugyo 120
samurai 58
Samyama 43, 84, 103
Sanmitsu 16, 57, 85, 105
Sanmitsu exercise 56
satisfaction 45, 46
satori 8–10, 13, 16, 17, 20, 29, 31–33, 42–44, 46, 48, 50, 58, 70, 72, 74, 75, 77, 80, 84, 88, 89, 91, 101, 102, 106, 108, 114, 116, 119–125, 141, 145, 146, 148, 149, 154–7, 159, 160
satori food 67
satori training 128, 132
sauna bath 135
secrets of longevity 51
Seishoku food 67
Seiza 104, 130
self-control 18–20, 79
self-correction 57
self-discovery 57, 71
self-healing 37, 54
self-improvement 29
self-knowledge 36
self-realizing 36
self-reference 114
self-reflection 74, 132
self-reliance 27, 37, 106

self-respect 45
Sendo 73
Sennin 32, 63, 73
Sermon on the Mount 45, 72
service 67
Shado 124
Shakuhachi 99
Shakya 26
Shambhava Mudra 101
Sharesmen 150
Shata Ataru 102
Shingaku 60
Shingon 34, 43, 85, 91, 116, 118, 130
Shingon-shu 32
Shingon Yuga 117
Shorinji Kempo 111
Shusei 96
Shuseiho 58, 77, 79, 132, 133
Shukkedo 70, 71
singing 79
sitting meditation 115
Siva 23
skepticism 40, 46
soba 68
soft living 82
Soto Zen 91, 116
spinal disorders 55
spiritual and moral sensivity 83
spiritual degeneracy 81
spiritual discipline 74, 153
spiritual exercises 72, 77, 81
spiritual training 19
stability 18, 53
stabilization 20
stamina method 88
stimulating hormone 56
strength 45
strengthening exercises 20
study 45, 47
suffering 92
Sufi 154
Sufi meditation 16

Index / 175

supernormal powers 21
suppuration 75
supreme selfishness 121
Sutras 18
Svetasvatara Upanisad 29
swinging movements 112
systematic nervous system 56, 92

Taittiriya 25
Tantric 81
Tao 73
T'ai Chi 111
T'an t'ien 53
tanden 53
Taoism 34, 73, 74, 77, 102
tapas 23, 24
tea-ceremony 135
telekinesis 91
temptations 123
Ten Commandments 43
Tendai 85, 117
Tenpu Nakamura Roshi 8
tension 52
theological discussion 35
Theravada Buddhism 102
thoracic breathing 55
three phases 83
Tibetan Buddhism 141
Tibetan esoteric Buddhism 117
tiredness 110
total attention 33
total organism 131
toxins 75
traditional dancing 135
true humanity 19
true love 95, 120
tuberclosis 142

Uddiyana 53
unbalanced diet 63
unconsciousness 90
unification 18, 37, 42, 86, 87
Upanisad 24, 28, 30, 37

Vaisesika 30
value judgments 84
Veda 23, 24
Vedanta 21, 22, 29
vegetarian 65
vigorous toweling 76
Vishnu 23
visualization 148
vitamins and minerals 64
Vow of *Kyokaho*, the 133
Vow of Meditation, the 136
Vow of Nutrition, the 134
Vow of Rest, the 136
Vow of *Shuseiho*, the 134

weak stomach 75
willingness 94
work training 120
worldly attachment 92
worldly thought 92
worship 45, 47, 74
worshipful mind 114
wrong diet 69

Yajur Veda 24
Yama 26, 42–45, 48
Yin and Yang 25, 41, 56, 90, 105
Yin-Yang philosophy 66
Yoga 14, 15, 29
Yoga Sutra 30, 43
Yoga training 89, 128
Yogasanas 49, 52–54, 56–58, 79, 100, 102
yoghurt 63
Yogic breathing 77, 112
Yogic Buddhism 83
Yogic food 65
Yogins 63, 65
Yogins 63, 84
Yomei School 60

Zazen 58, 69, 70, 75, 80, 92, 105, 106, 115, 116, 137, 148, 153

Zen 17, 32, 34, 41, 49–51, 58, 74, 78, 82, 88, 90, 92, 103, 110, 120, 128, 131, 140–142, 153
Zen *Koan* 101
Zen-shu 74
Zen training 17

Zengyo 49, 106, 115
Zenteki 110
Zesshoku 74, 75
Zoroaster 33
Zoroastrianism 149